Birgit Zirn · Karl Mehnert *Eds.*

Guide for
Genetic Consultation

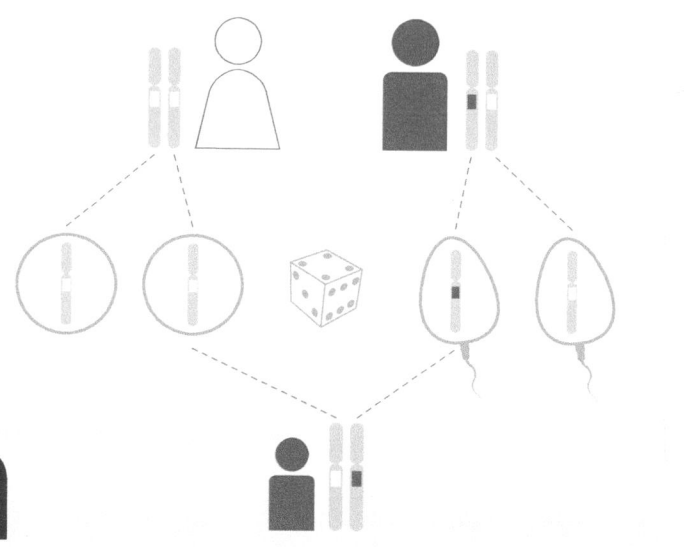

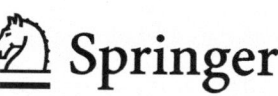 Springer

Authors:

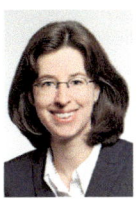

Prof. Dr. Dr. med. Birgit Zirn (Stuttgart) is a specialist in medical genetics and director of genetikum® Stuttgart.
After obtaining degrees in medicine, biology and musicology, Prof. Zirn completed her clinical and academic training in human genetics and paediatrics with syndromology as a specialist subject. Birgit Zirn developed and presented the graphics contained in this manual in talks and lectures.

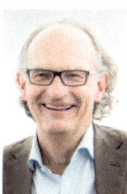

Dr. med. Karl Mehnert (Neu-Ulm) is the founder and chief medical officer of genetikum®, a medical institution offering genetic counselling and diagnostics in a number of locations in Southern Germany.
Having completed a medical degree and further training in clinical genetics at the University of Ulm, Dr. Mehnert set up in Neu-Ulm in 1990 as an expert in medical genetics and founded the genetikum®. Karl Mehnert contributed expertise accumulated in 25 years of genetic counselling to this manual.

Implementation, layout and design:
Dr. rer. nat. Petra Freilinger, MBA, genetikum®, Neu-Ulm, Germany
Dr. med. Claus Münster, Remy & Remy Gesundheitskommunikation GmbH, Augsburg, Germany

Produced in collaboration with the following genetikum® staff members:
Dr. med. Gabriele du Bois, Dr. med. Anna Lena Burgemeister, Dr. rer. nat. Eva Daumiller, Dr. rer. physiol. Ilona Dietze-Armana, Dr. rer. nat. Petra Freilinger, Dr. med. Harald Gaspar, Dr. biol. hum. Andreas Gerhardinger, Prof. Dr. med. Horst Hameister, Dr. med. Silke Hartmann, Dr. med. Alina Henn, PD Dr. med. Wolfram Klein, Dr. biol. hum. Marius Kuhn, Dr. med. Verena Pfaff, Dr. biol. hum. Günther Rettenberger, Dr. Eva Rossier, Dr. med. Maren Wenzel

ISBN 978-3-030-04344-5
ISBN 978-3-030-04345-2 (ebook)
DOI 10.1007/978-3-030-04345-2

Library of Congress Control Number: 2019934474

Translation from the German language edition: *Handbuch für die Genetische Sprechstunde* by Birgit Zirn and Karl Mehnert, © Springer-Verlag 2017. All Rights Reserved.

This Springer imprint is published by the registered company Springer Nature Switzerland AG
The registered company address is: Gewerbestrasse 11, 6330 Cham, Switzerland

Guide for Genetic Consultation
Contents

A Basic Principles

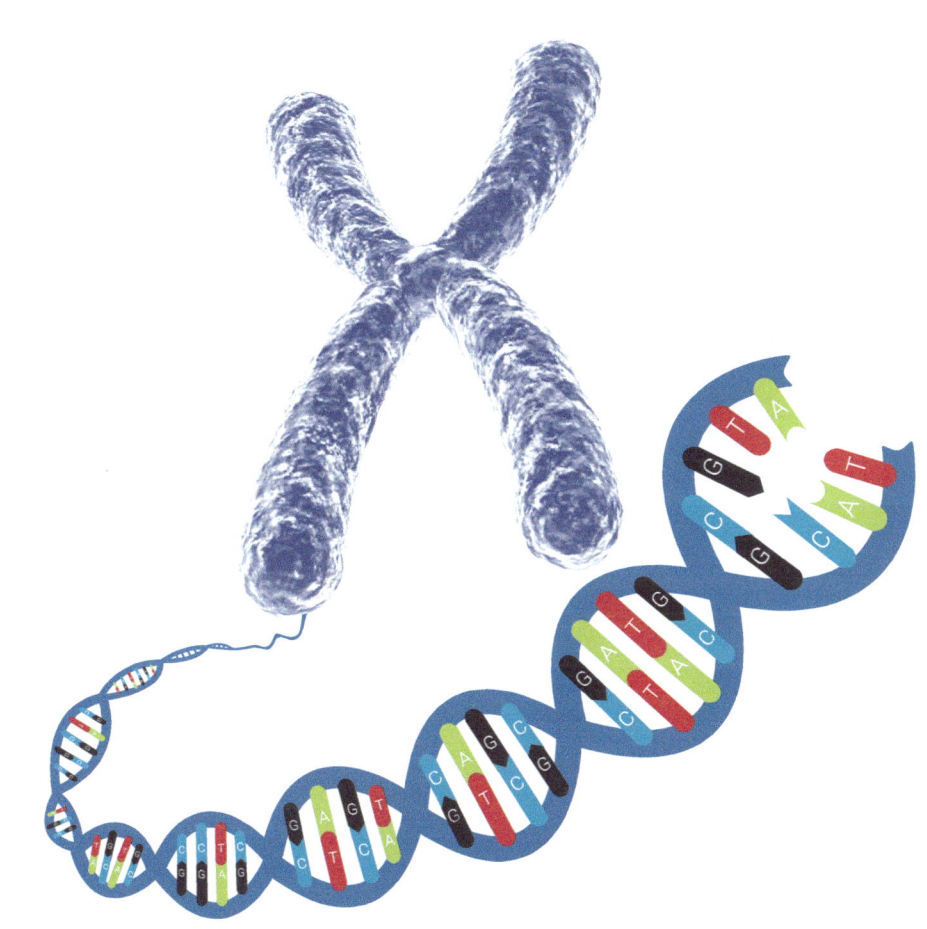

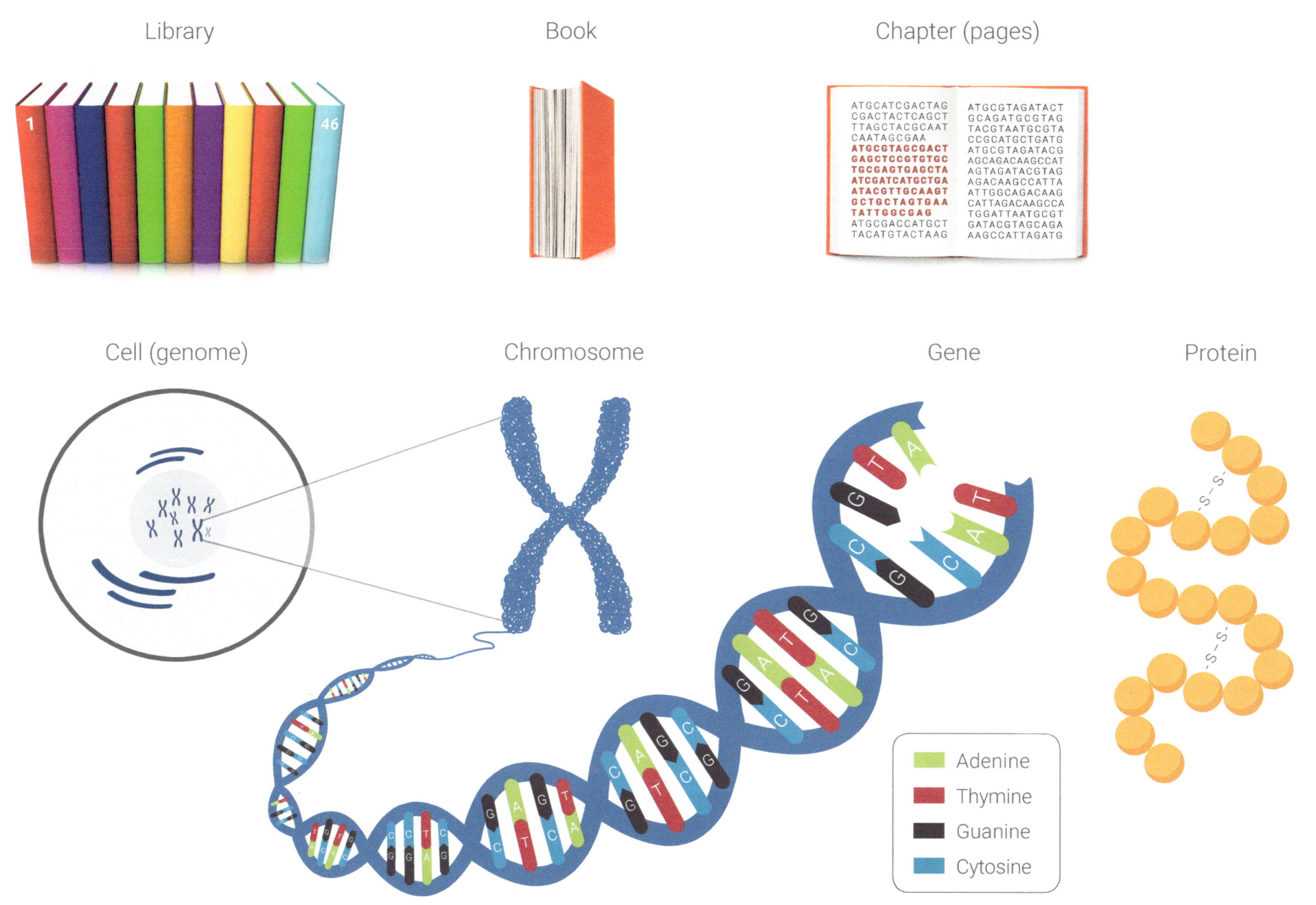

Library

Book

Chapter (pages)

Cell (genome)

Chromosome

Gene

Protein

Adenine
Thymine
Guanine
Cytosine

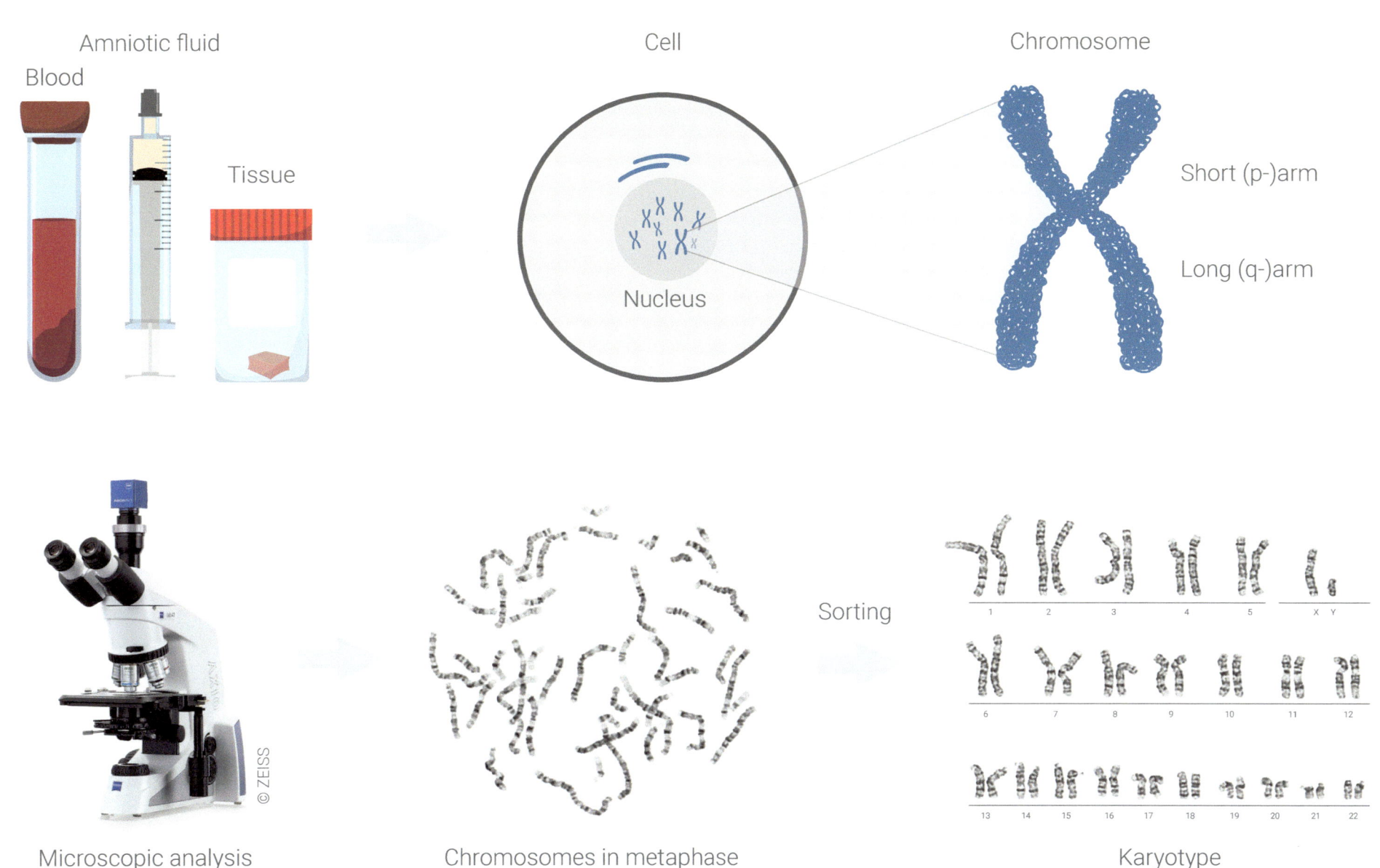

Blood

Amniotic fluid

Tissue

Cell

Nucleus

Chromosome

Short (p-)arm

Long (q-)arm

Microscopic analysis
Resolution approx. 5–10 Mb

Chromosomes in metaphase

Sorting

Karyotype

FISH = **f**luorescent **in s**itu **h**ybridisation

Normal result

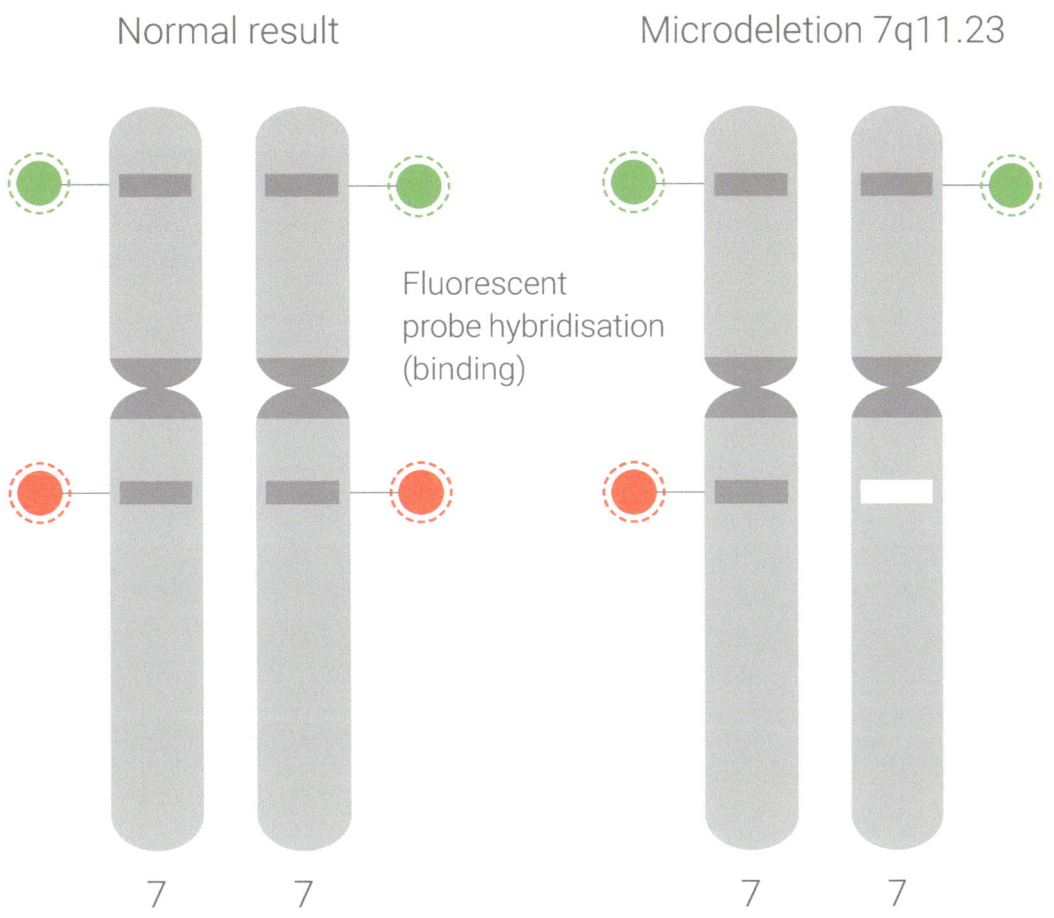

Fluorescent probe hybridisation (binding)

7   7

Microdeletion 7q11.23

7   7

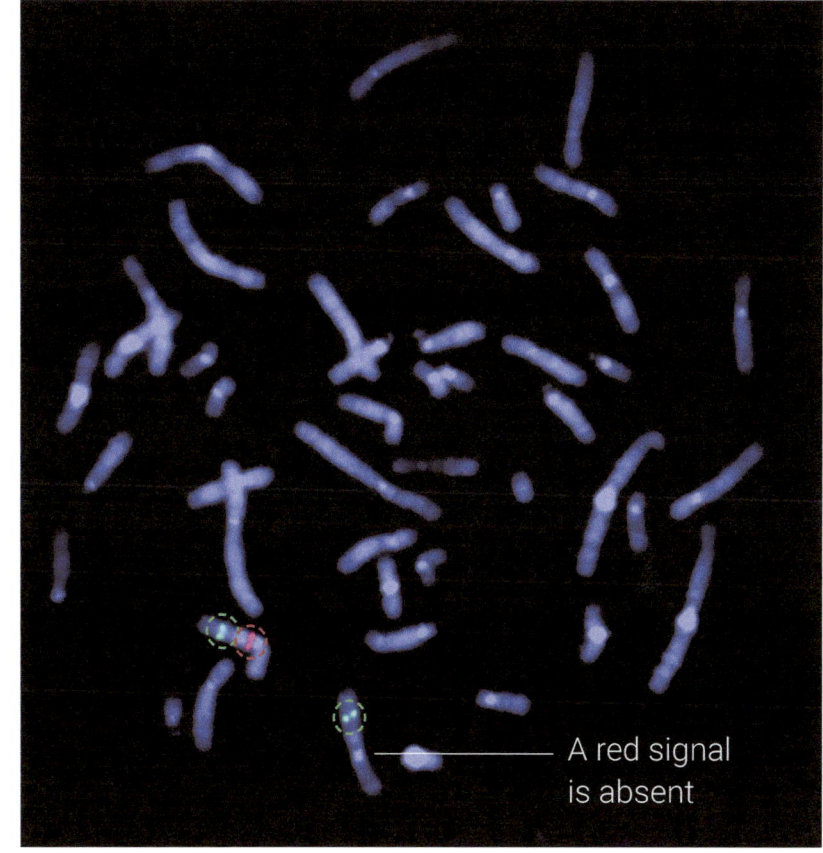

A red signal is absent

Microdeletion 7q11.23 manifests clinically as Williams syndrome

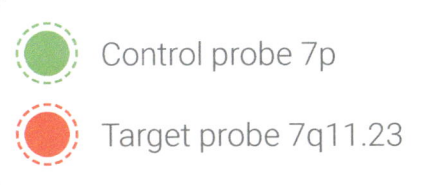

- ● Control probe 7p
- ● Target probe 7q11.23

Array CGH = array comparative genomic hybridisation

Molecular karyotyping (high-resolution chromosome analysis) identifies microdeletions and microduplications

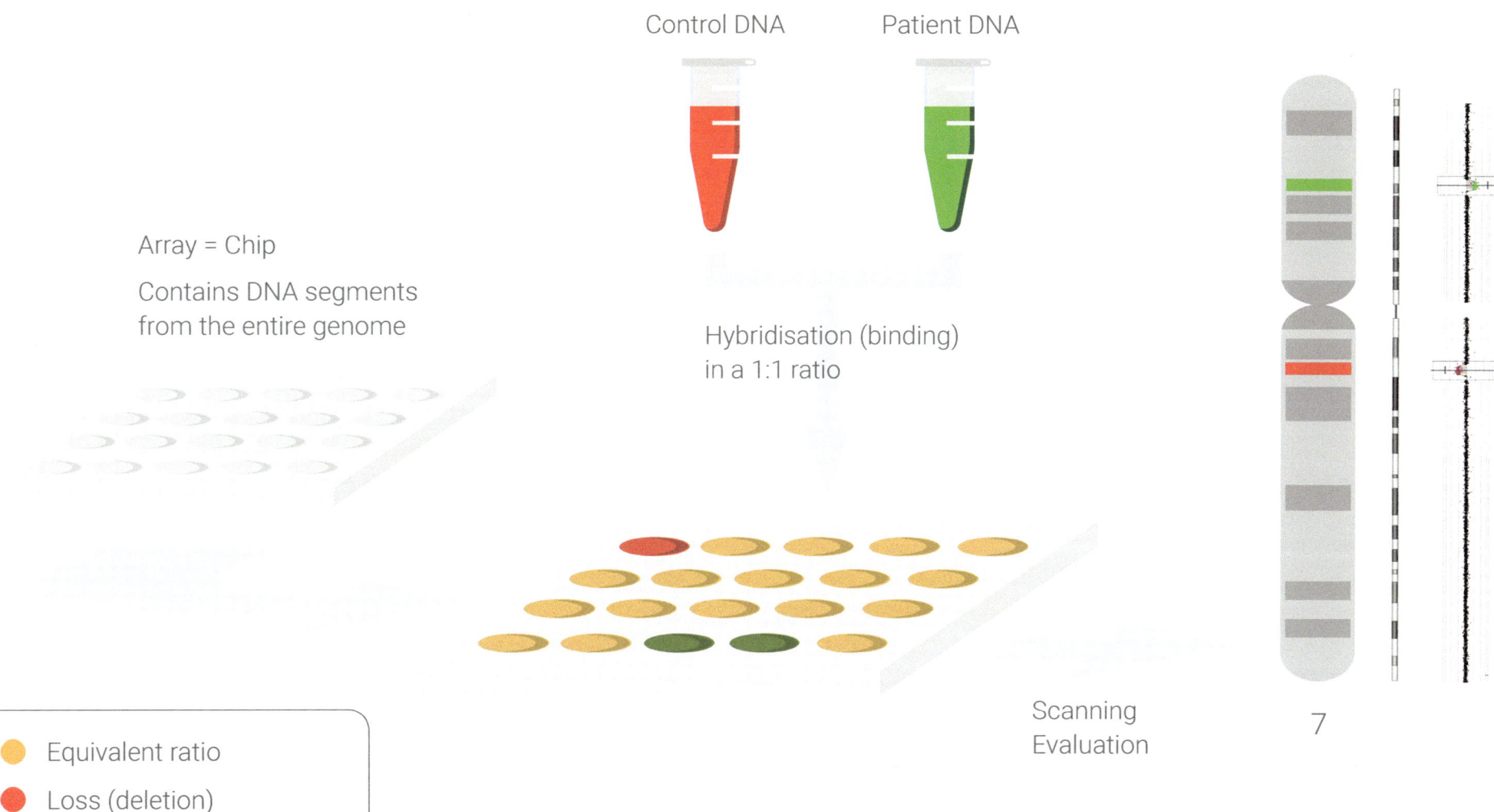

Control DNA

Patient DNA

Array = Chip

Contains DNA segments from the entire genome

Hybridisation (binding) in a 1:1 ratio

Scanning Evaluation

7

Equivalent ratio

Loss (deletion)

Gain (duplication)

Array comparative genomic hybridisation = high-resolution chromosome analysis

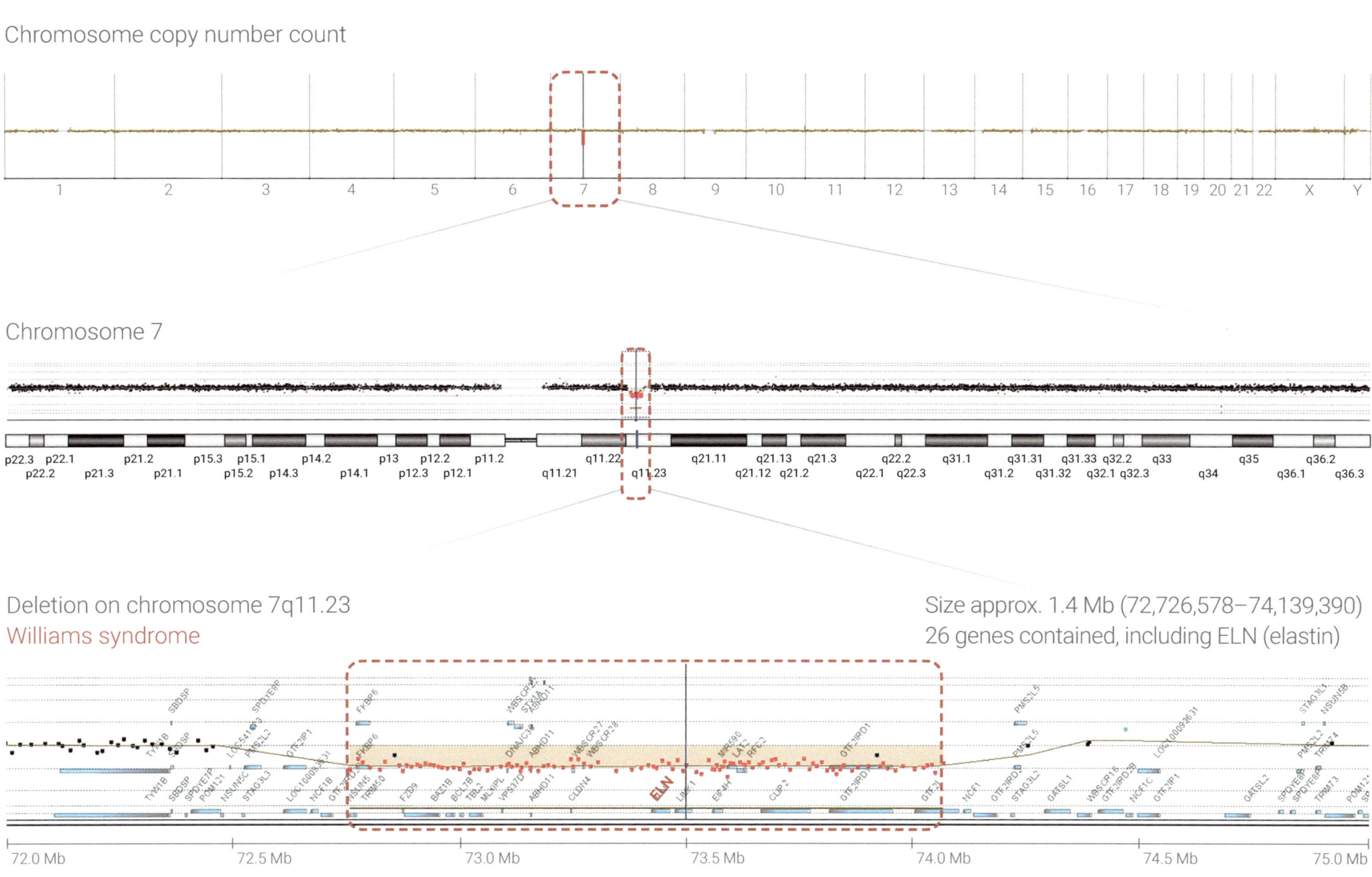

Chromosome copy number count

Chromosome 7

Deletion on chromosome 7q11.23
Williams syndrome

Size approx. 1.4 Mb (72,726,578–74,139,390)
26 genes contained, including ELN (elastin)

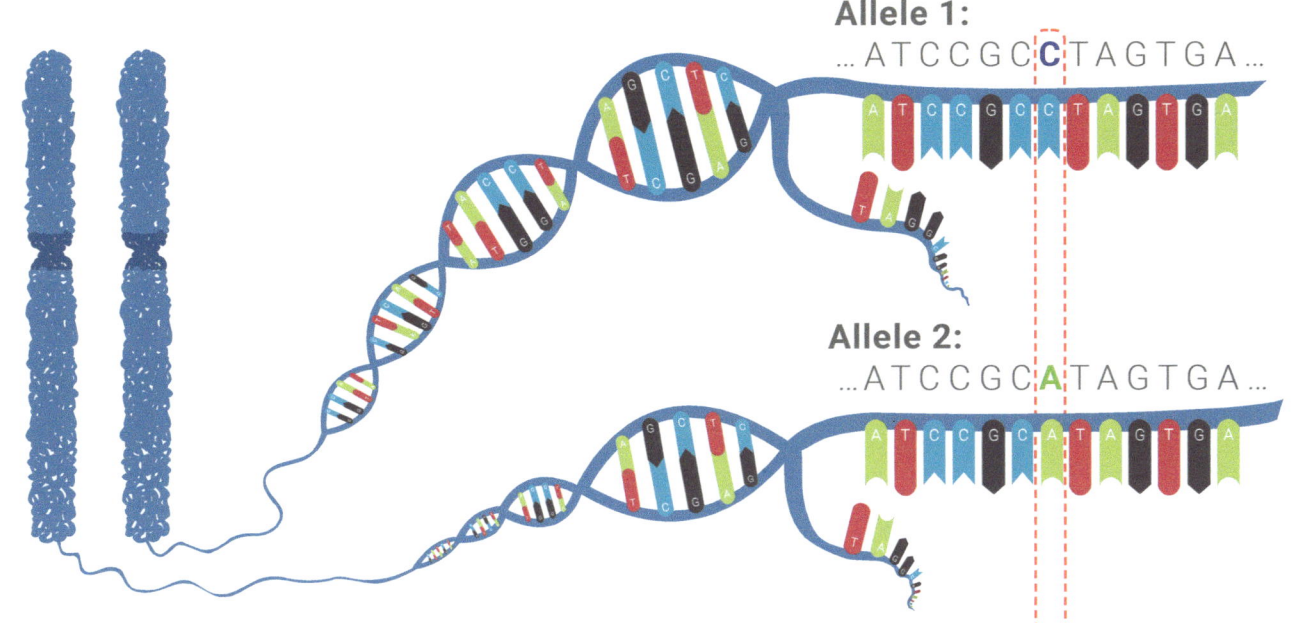

Allele 1:
... A T C C G C **C** T A G T G A ...

Allele 2:
... A T C C G C **A** T A G T G A ...

Reference	A T C C G C **C** T A G T G A	Reference	A T C C G C **C** T A G T G A	Reference	A T C C G C **C** T A G T G A
Allele 1	A T C C G C **C** T A G T G A	**Allele 1**	A T C C G C **C** T A G T G A	**Allele 1**	A T C C G C **A** T A G T G A
Allele 2	A T C C G C **C** T A G T G A	**Allele 2**	A T C C G C **A** T A G T G A	**Allele 2**	A T C C G C **A** T A G T G A

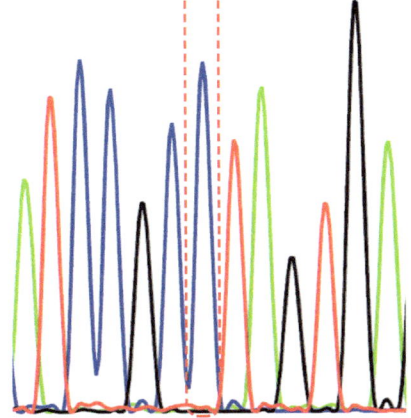

Normal sequence

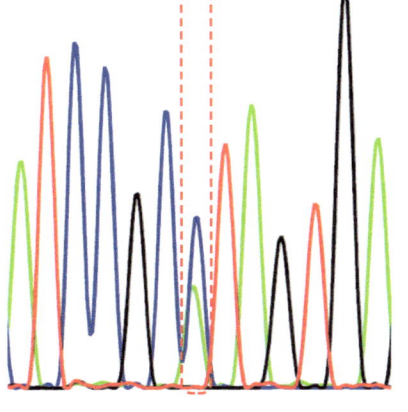

Heterozygous mutation

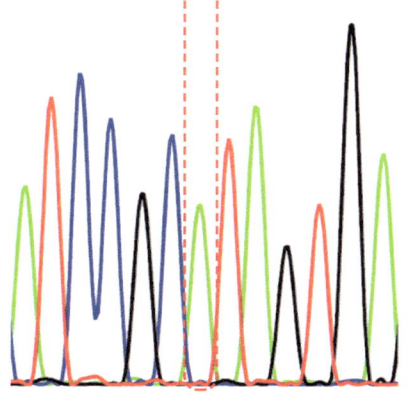

Homozygous mutation

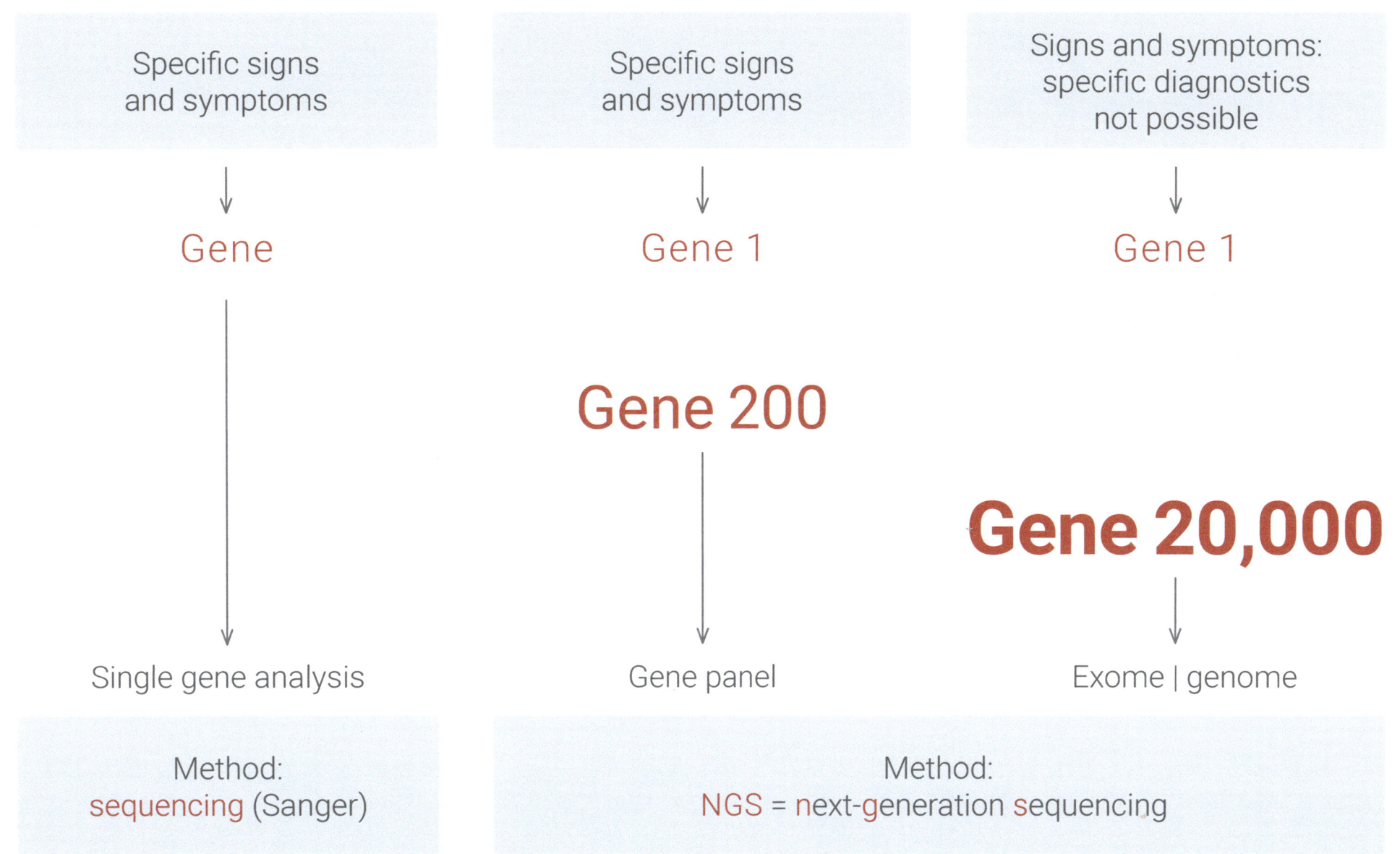

B Cytogenetics

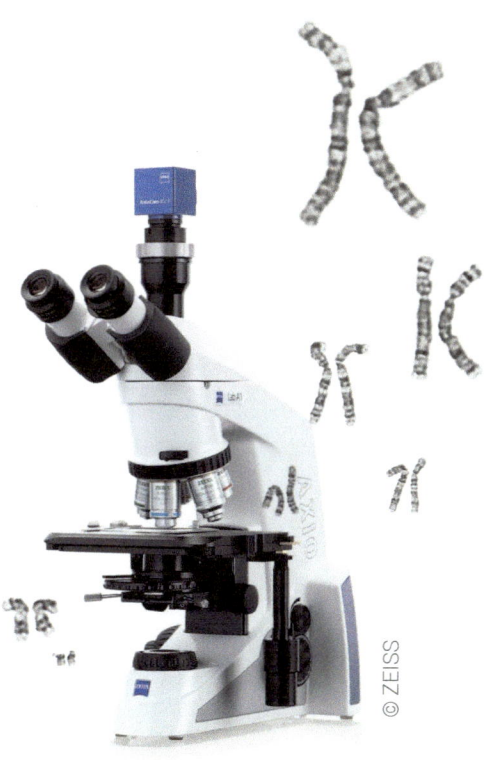

© ZEISS

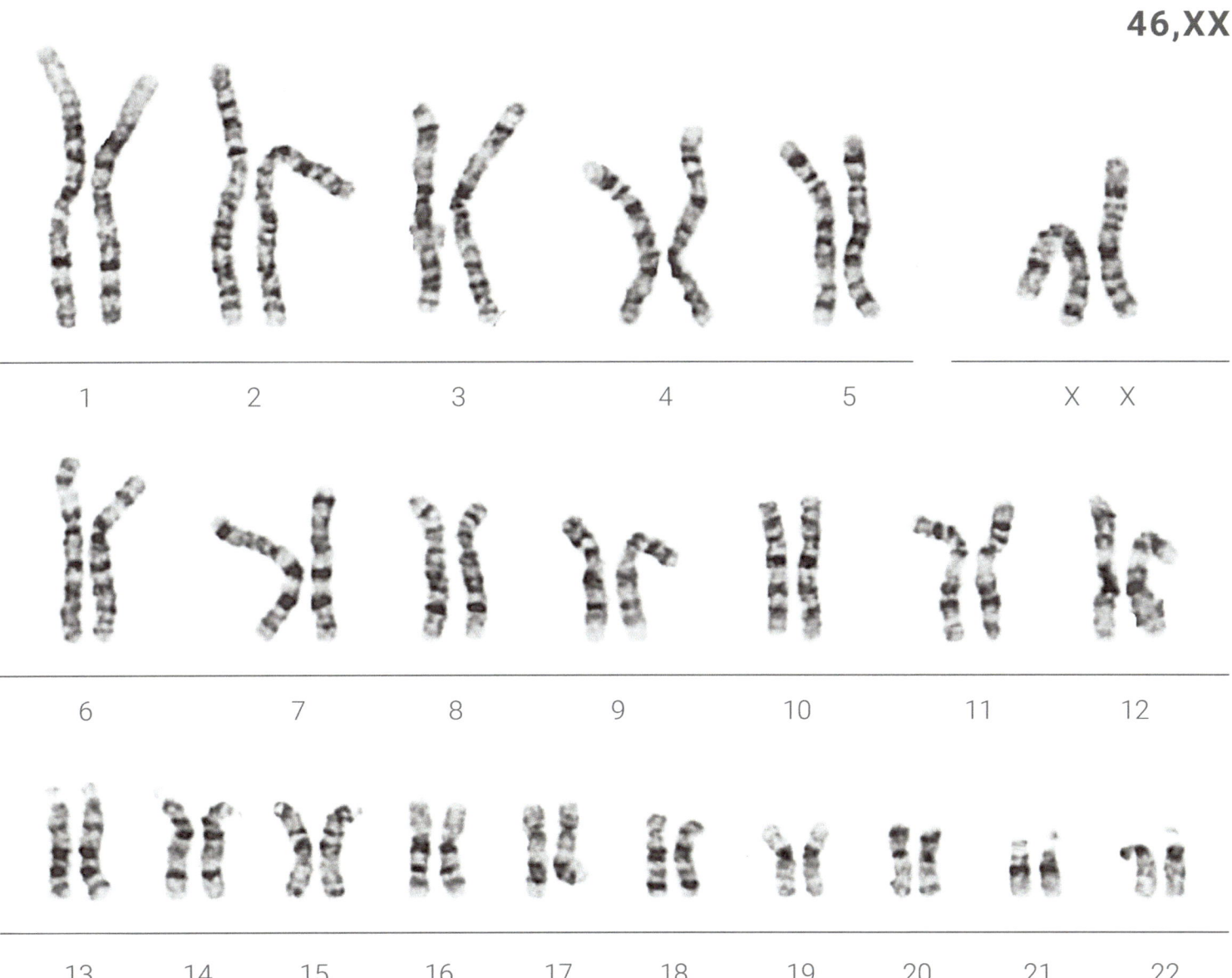

46,XY

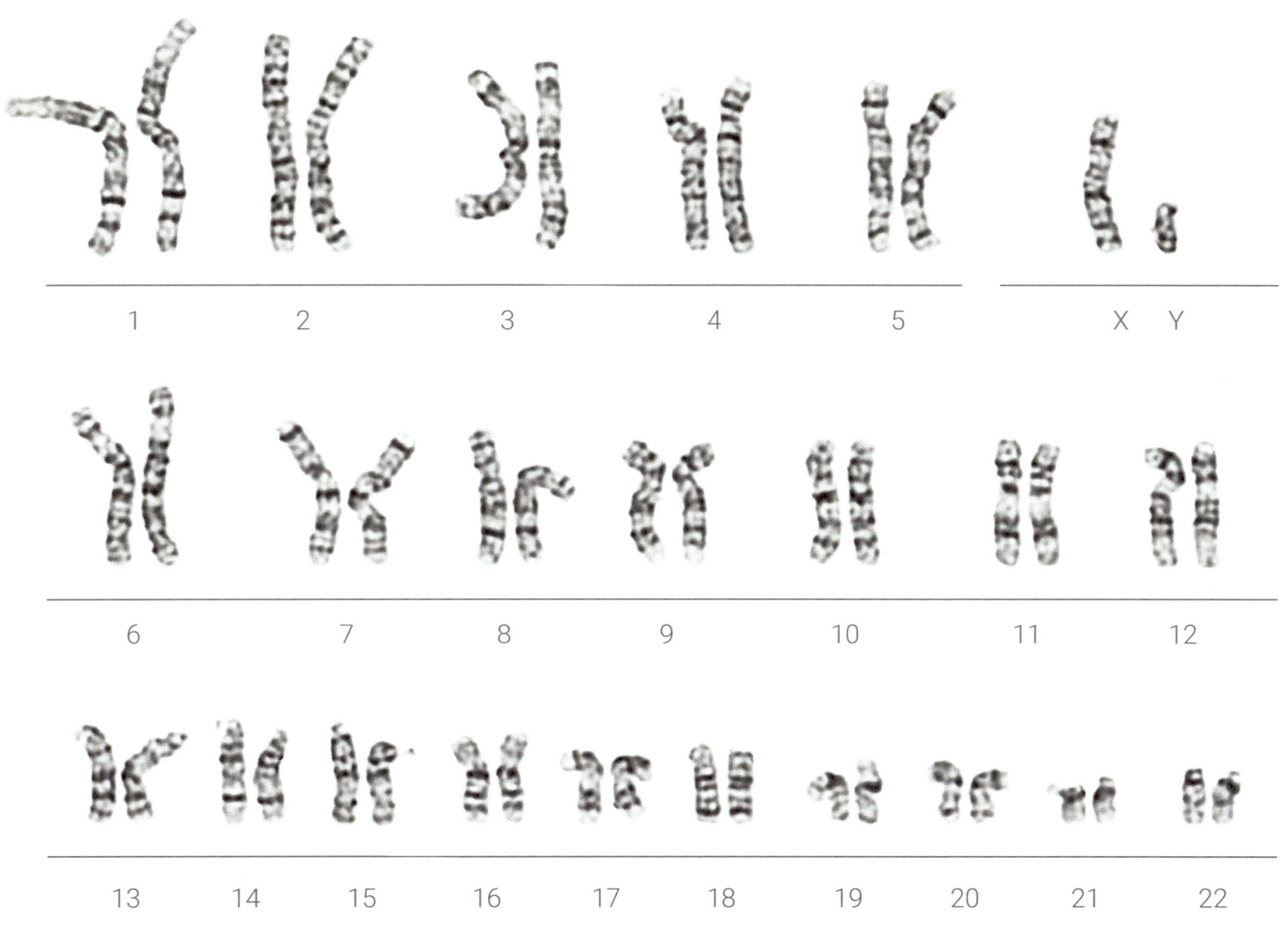

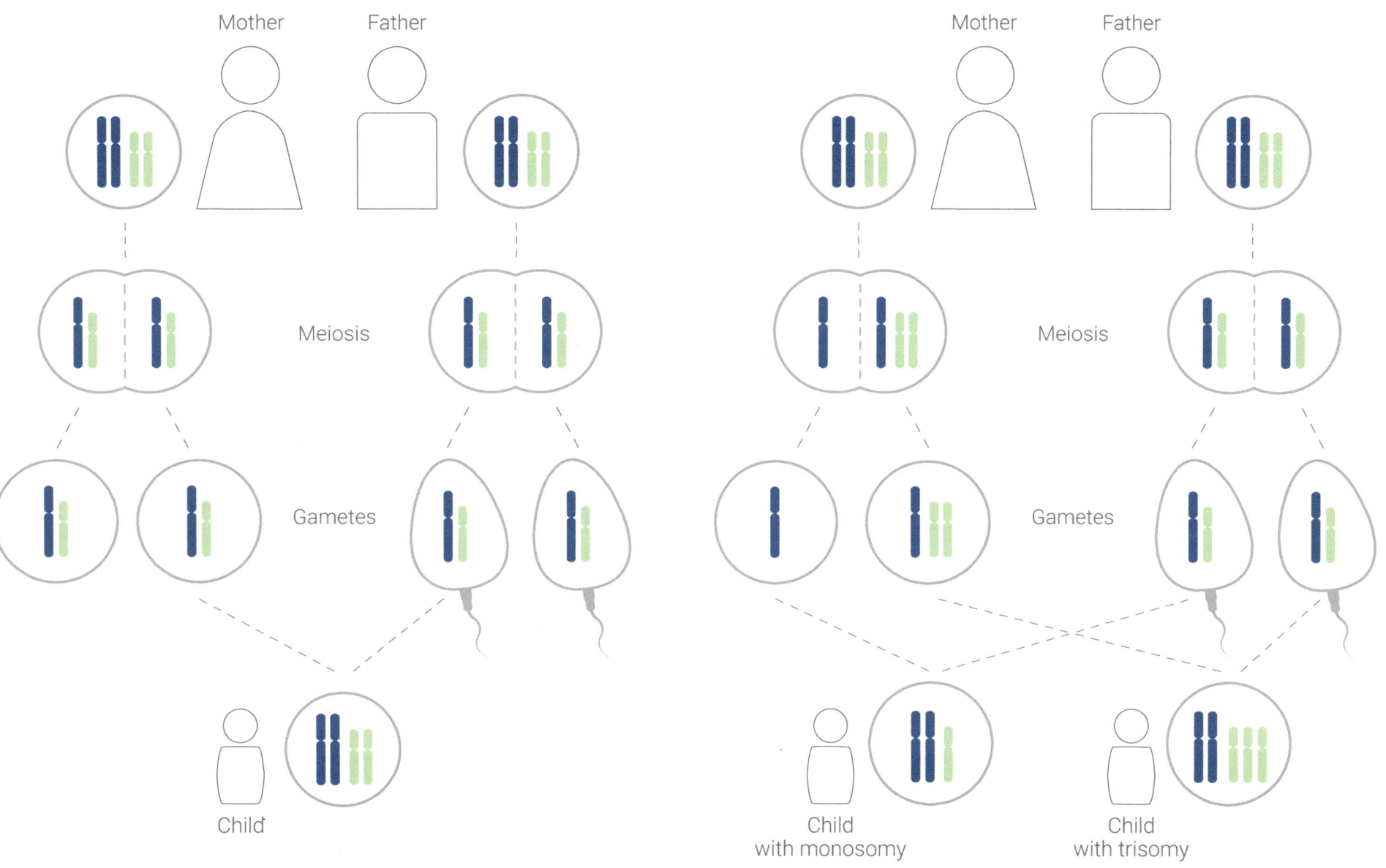

Normal gamete formation

Mother   Father

Meiosis

Gametes

Child

Nondisjunction

Mother   Father

Meiosis

Gametes

Child with monosomy   Child with trisomy

47,XX,+21

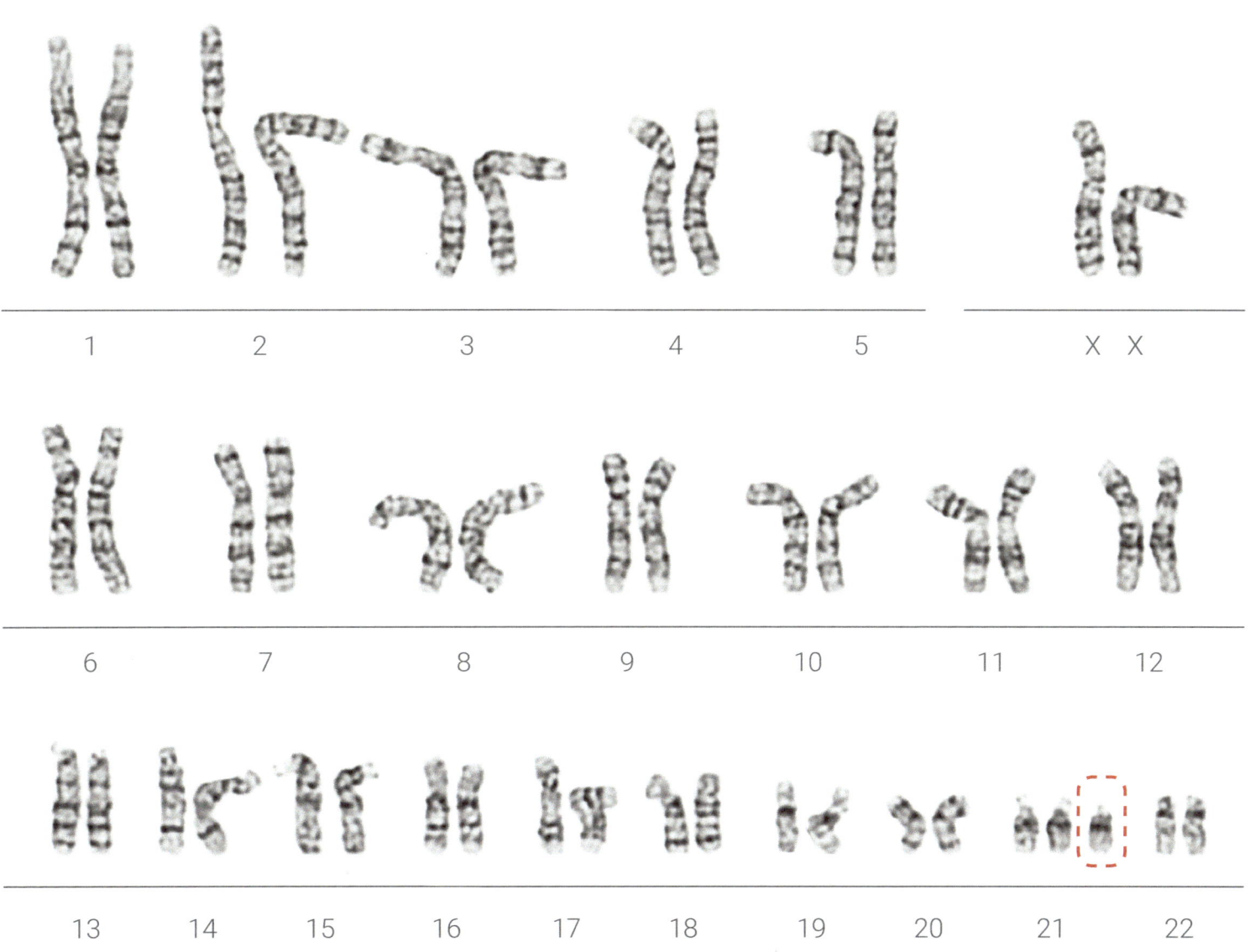

Nondisjunction in maternal meiosis

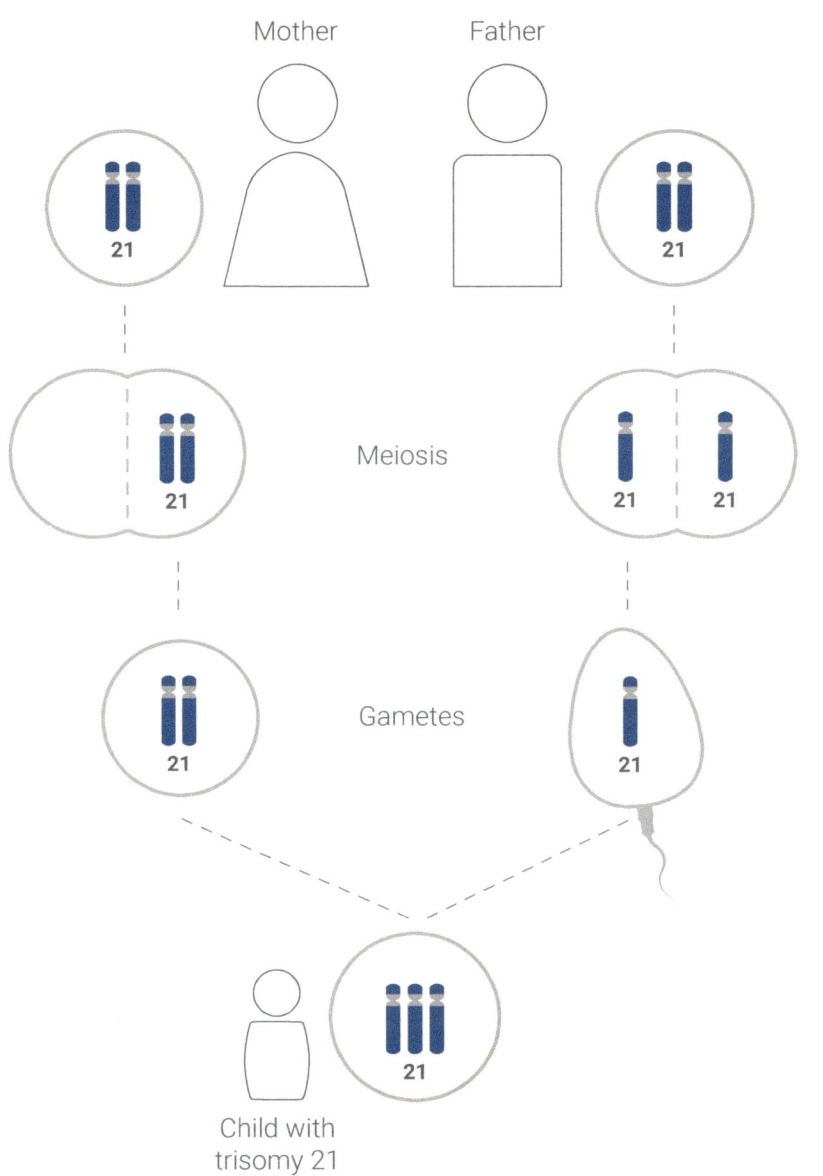

Mother

Father

Meiosis

Gametes

21

21

21

21

21

21

21

21

Child with
trisomy 21

21

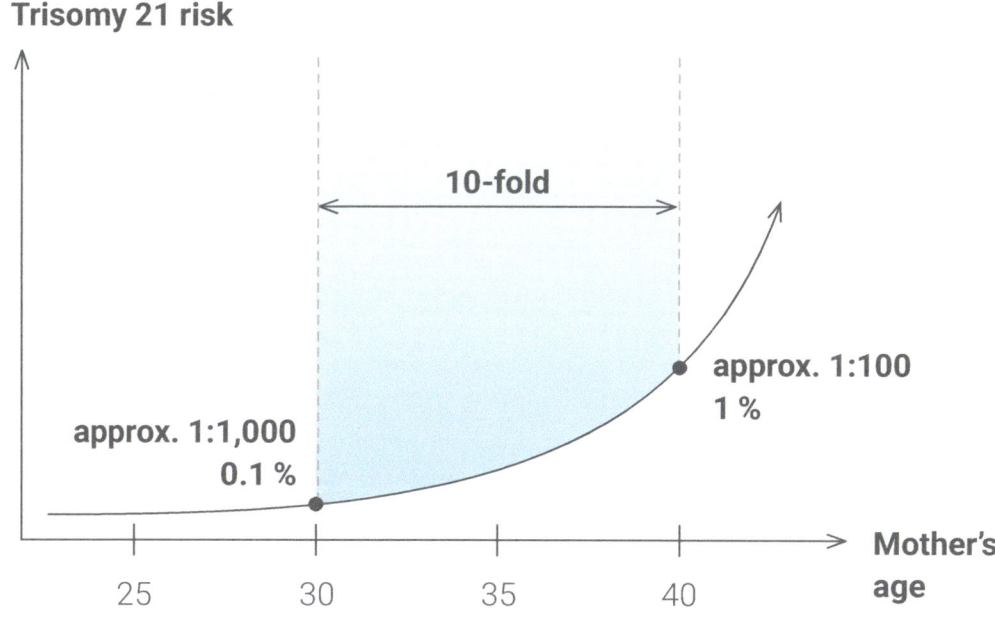

Trisomy 21 risk

10-fold

approx. 1:100
1 %

approx. 1:1,000
0.1 %

25   30   35   40

**Mother's
age**

Son: Translocation trisomy 21
46,XY,der(14;21)(q10;q10),+21

Father: Healthy carrier of a Robertsonian translocation
45,XY,der(14;21)(q10;q10)

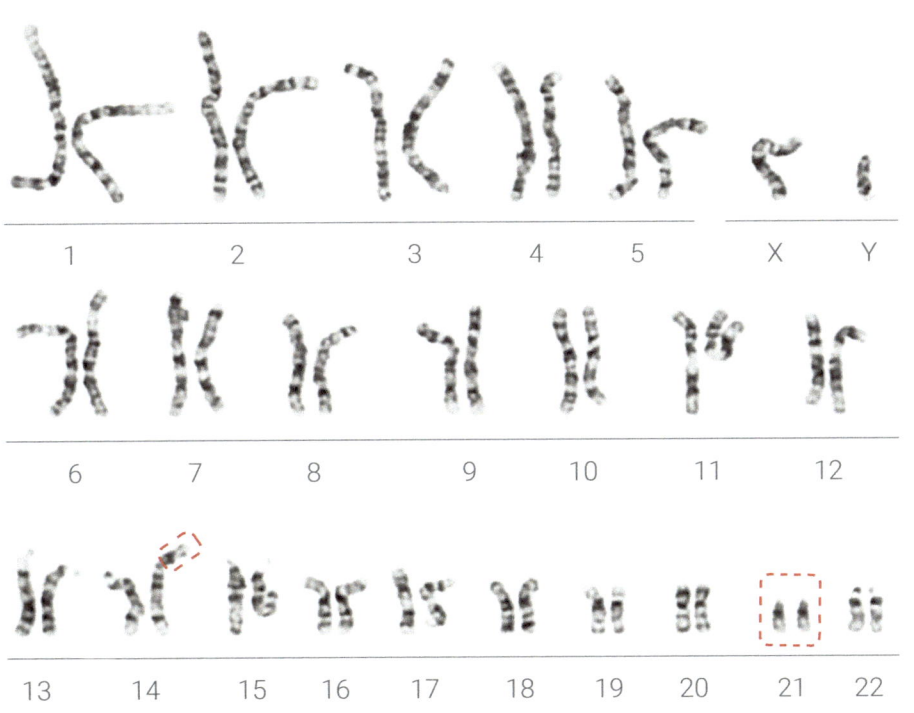

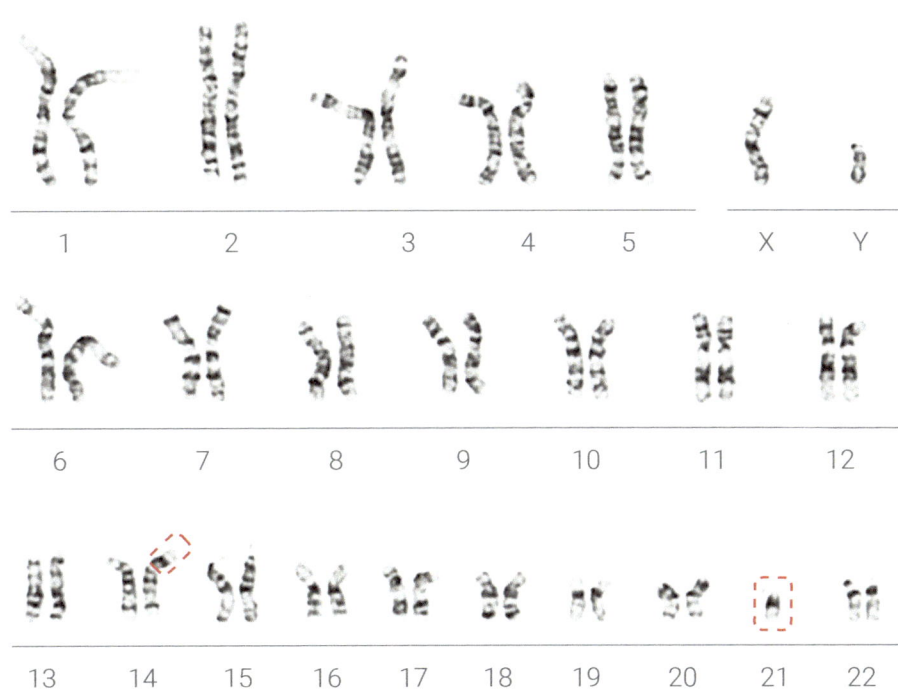

Incidence:

1:700

95 % trisomy 21 with an additional chromosome 21

5 % translocation trisomy 21

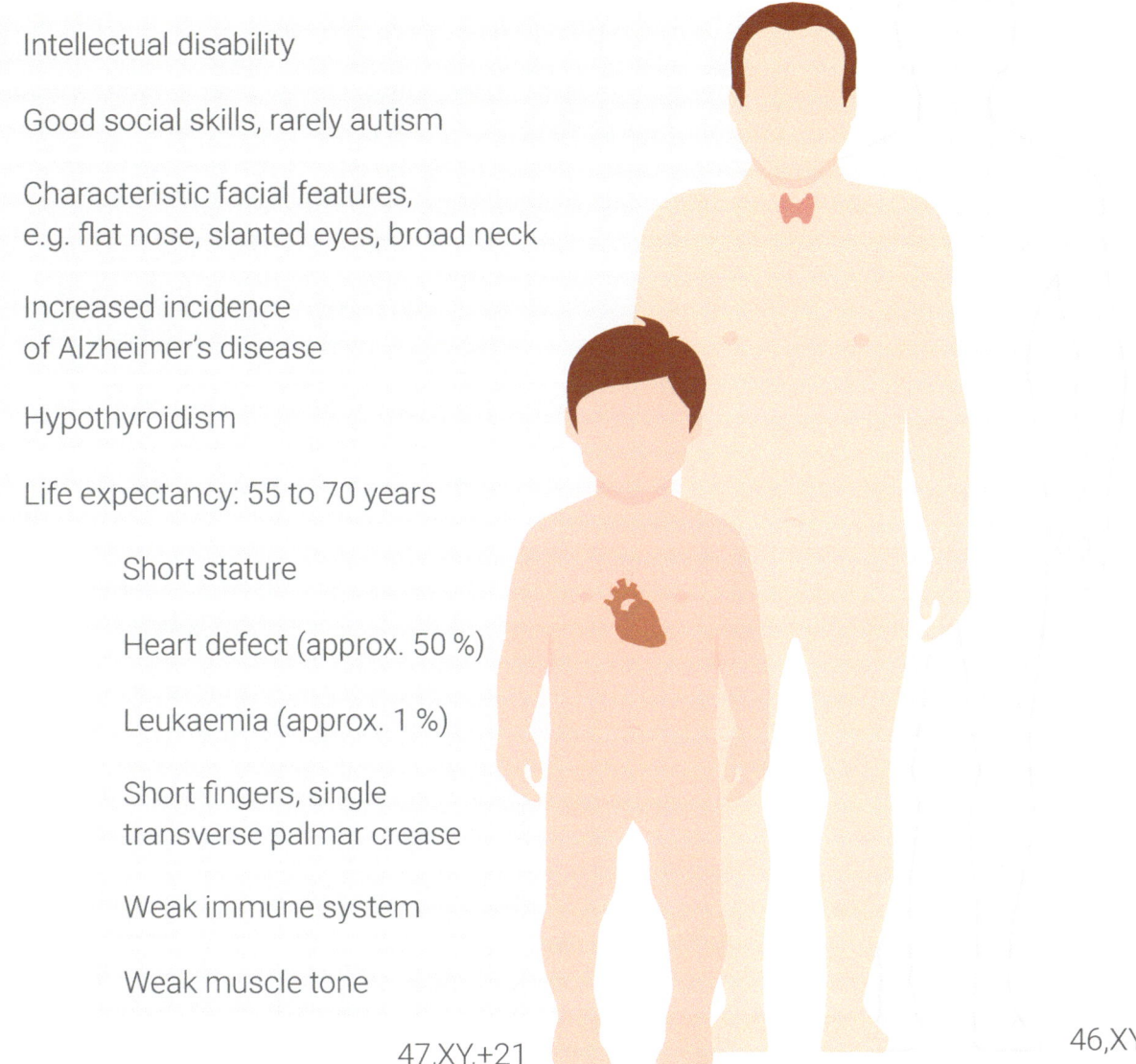

Intellectual disability

Good social skills, rarely autism

Characteristic facial features,
e.g. flat nose, slanted eyes, broad neck

Increased incidence
of Alzheimer's disease

Hypothyroidism

Life expectancy: 55 to 70 years

Short stature

Heart defect (approx. 50 %)

Leukaemia (approx. 1 %)

Short fingers, single
transverse palmar crease

Weak immune system

Weak muscle tone

47,XY,+21   46,XY

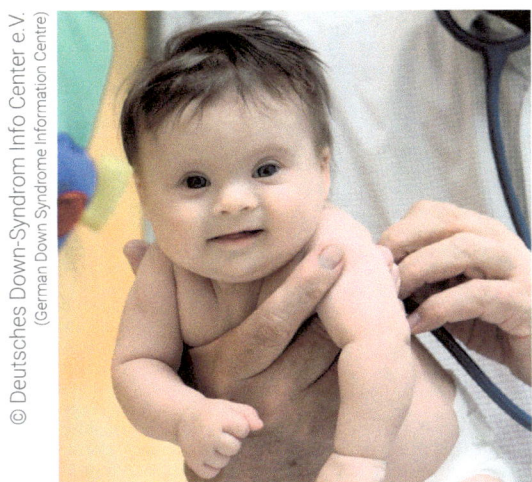

Girl (3 months) with
Down syndrome (47,XX,+21)

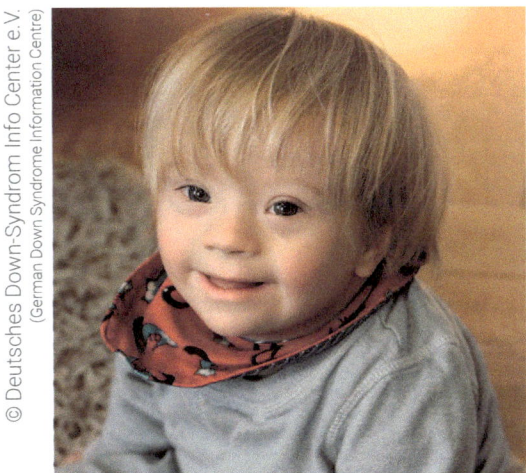

Boy (18 months) with
Down syndrome (47,XY,+21)

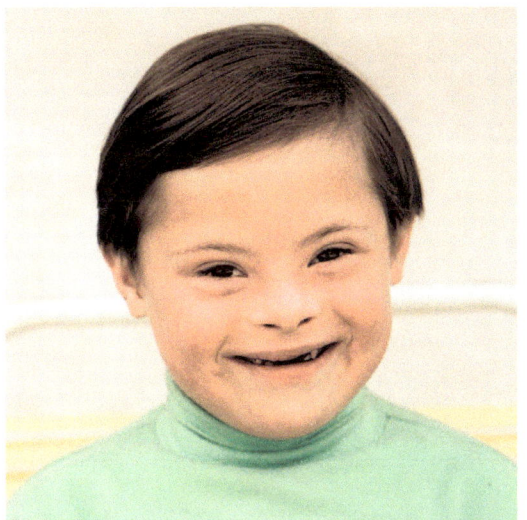

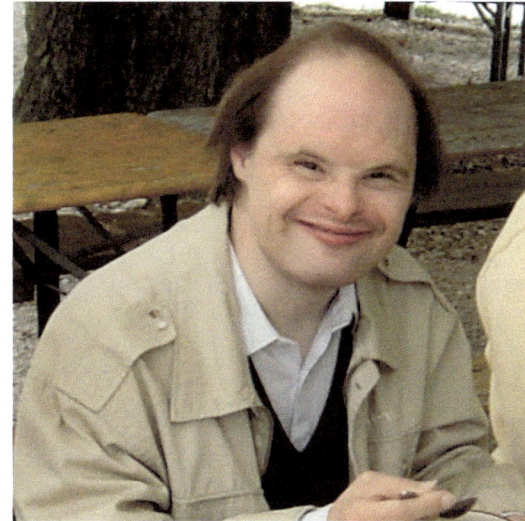

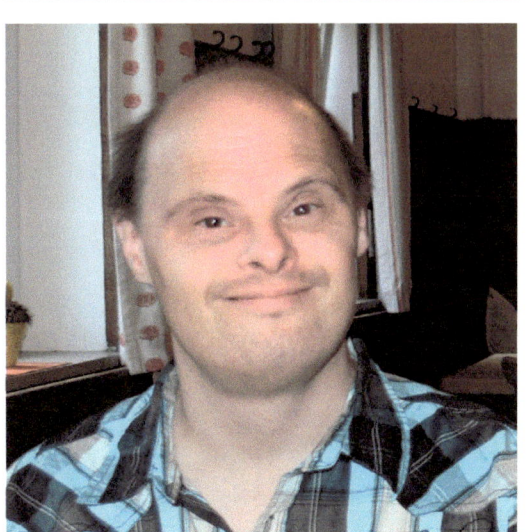

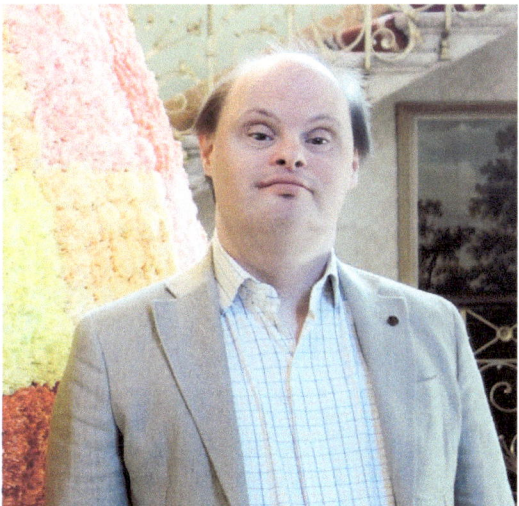

Boy/man with Down syndrome (47,XY,+21)
at the ages of 7, 40 and 50 (bottom row of pictures)

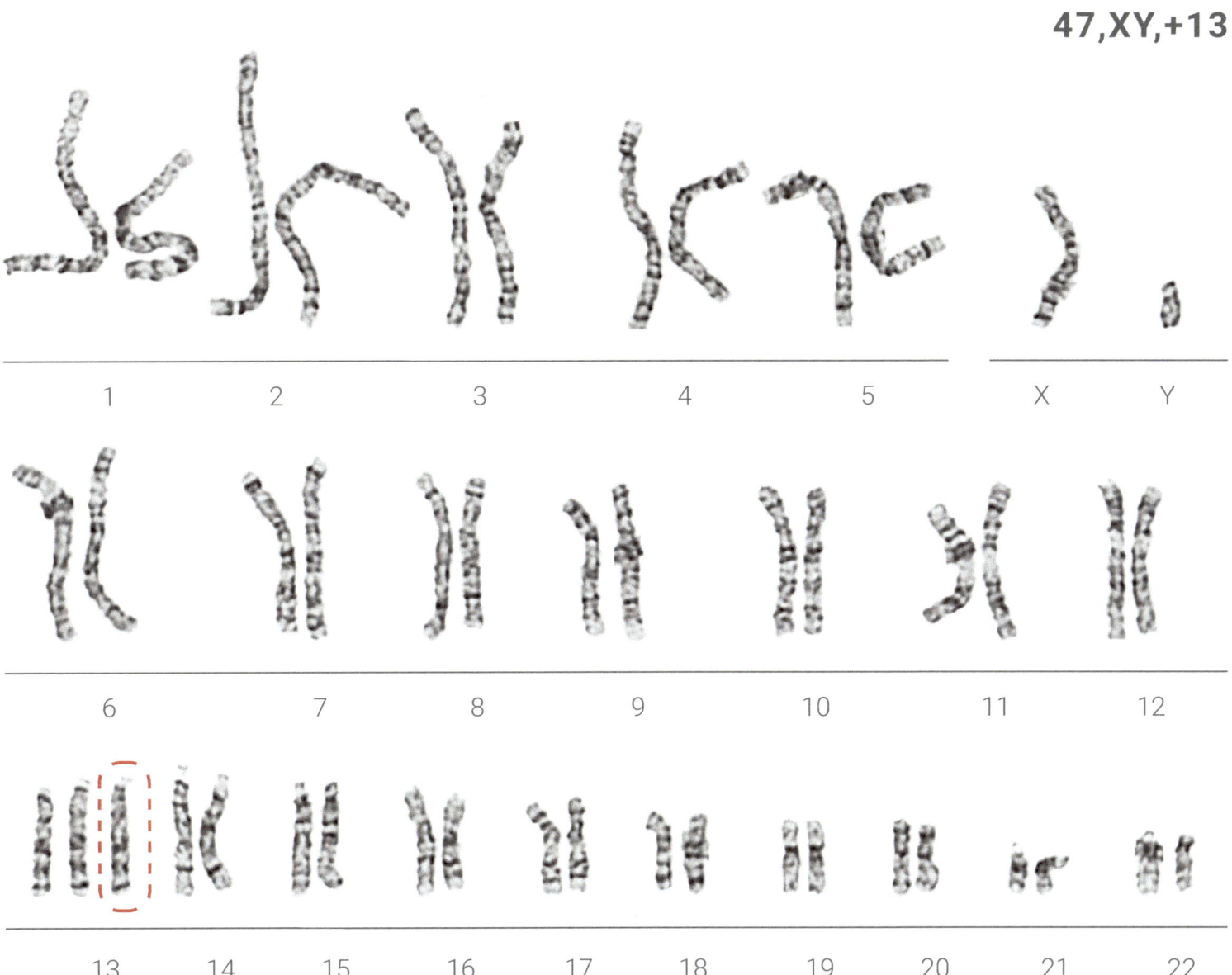

47,XY,+13

| 1 | 2 | 3 | 4 | 5 | X | Y |

| 6 | 7 | 8 | 9 | 10 | 11 | 12 |

| 13 | 14 | 15 | 16 | 17 | 18 | 19 | 20 | 21 | 22 |

47,XX,+18

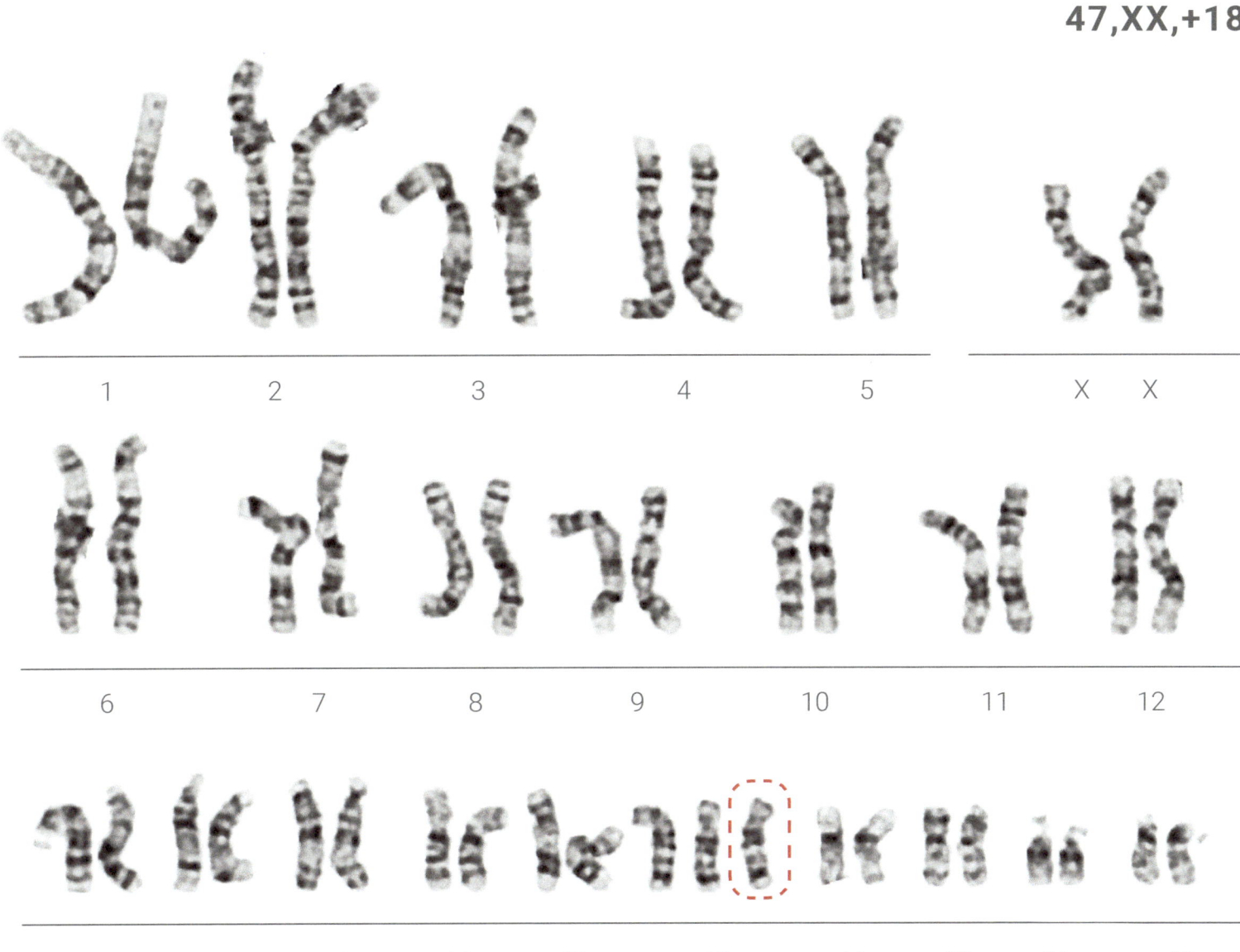

Shared characteristics of trisomies 13 and 18:

• Frequent pregnancy loss (80–90 %)
• Prenatal growth deficiency (small embryo, small head)
• Severe malformations (heart, brain, kidneys)
• Low life expectancy, severe developmental disorder

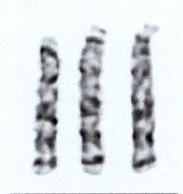

13

**Trisomy 13
Pätau syndrome
Incidence 1:8,000**

Additional features:

Cleft lip/palate

Extra fingers (polydactyly)

Holoprosencephaly

Eye anomalies

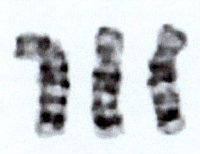

18

**Trisomy 18
Edwards syndrome
Incidence 1:6,000**

Additional features:

Omphalocele

Prominent back portion of the head

Finger overlap

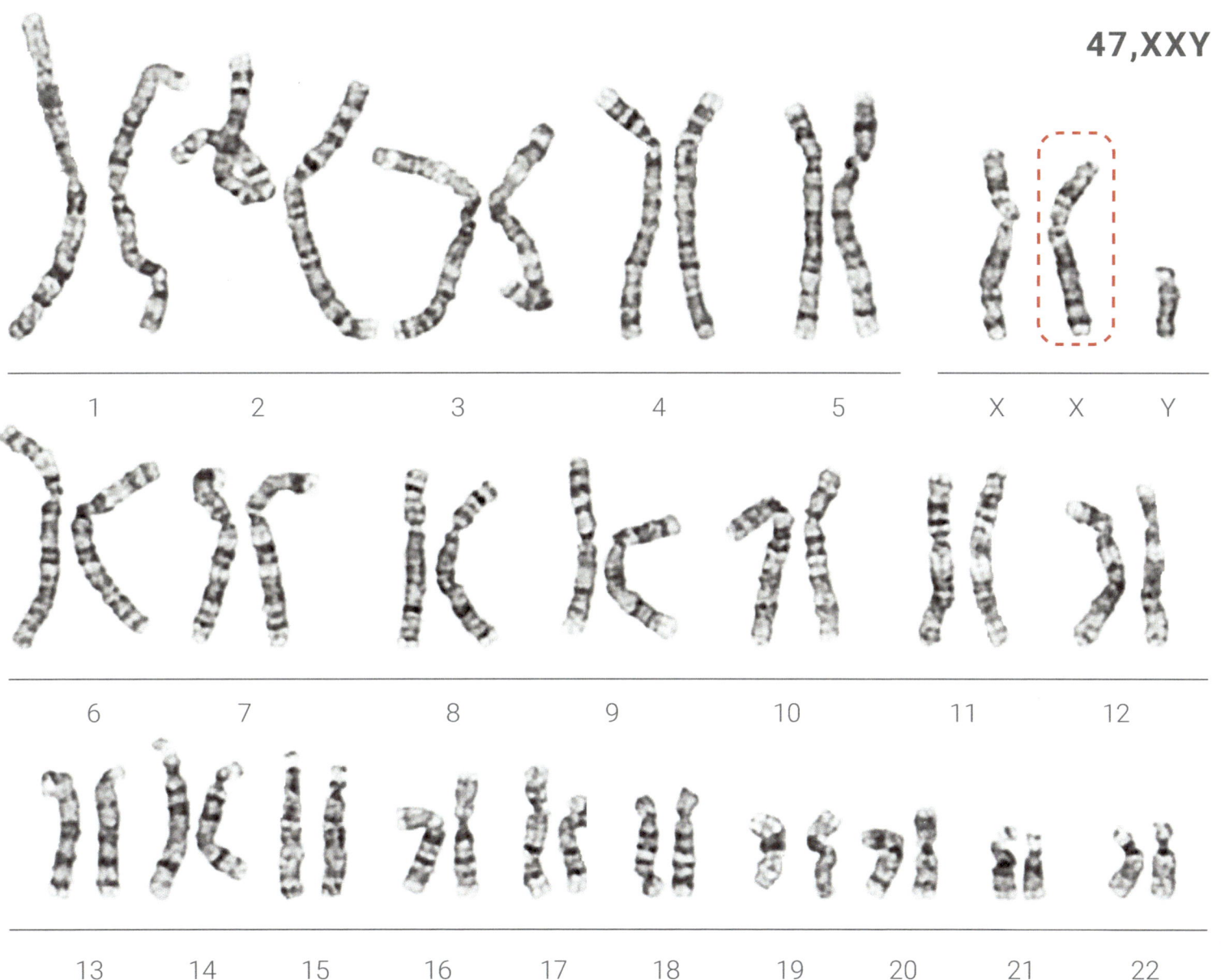

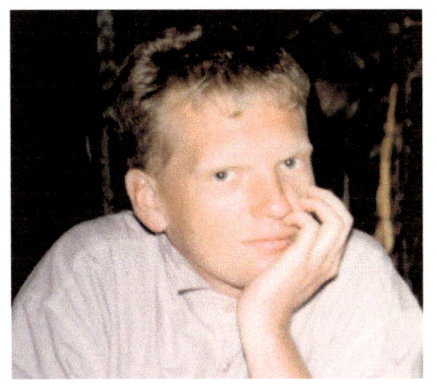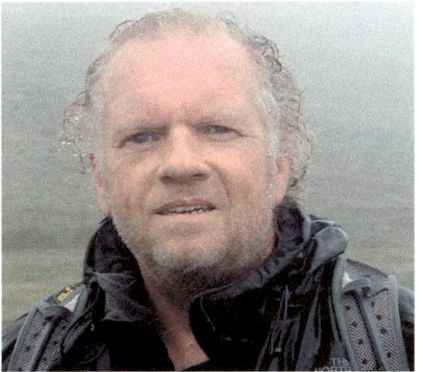

Man (at ages 23 and 54 years) with Klinefelter syndrome (47,XXY)

Incidence:

1:500 bis 1:1,000 (boys/men)

Therapy:

Testosterone

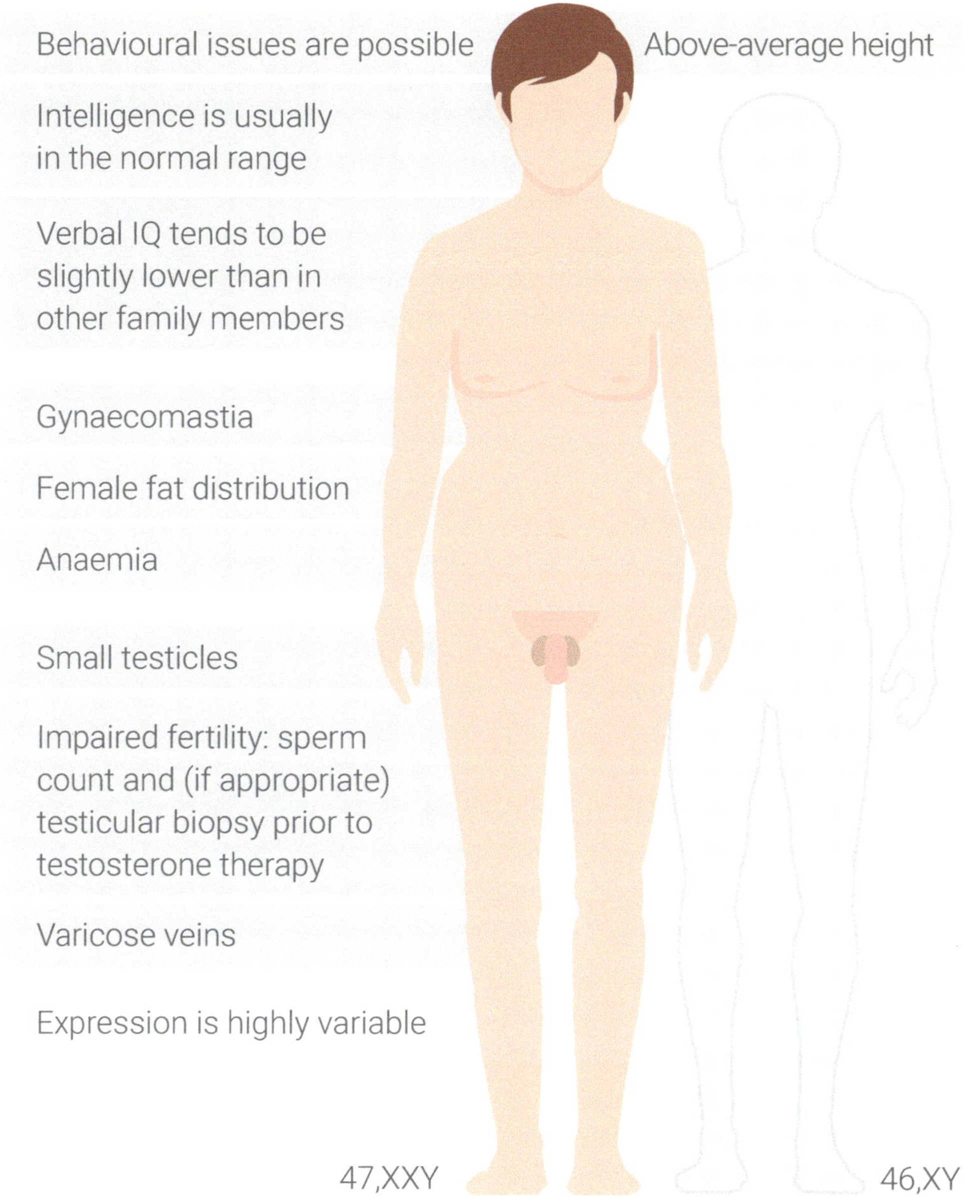

Behavioural issues are possible

Above-average height

Intelligence is usually in the normal range

Verbal IQ tends to be slightly lower than in other family members

Gynaecomastia

Female fat distribution

Anaemia

Small testicles

Impaired fertility: sperm count and (if appropriate) testicular biopsy prior to testosterone therapy

Varicose veins

Expression is highly variable

47,XXY

46,XY

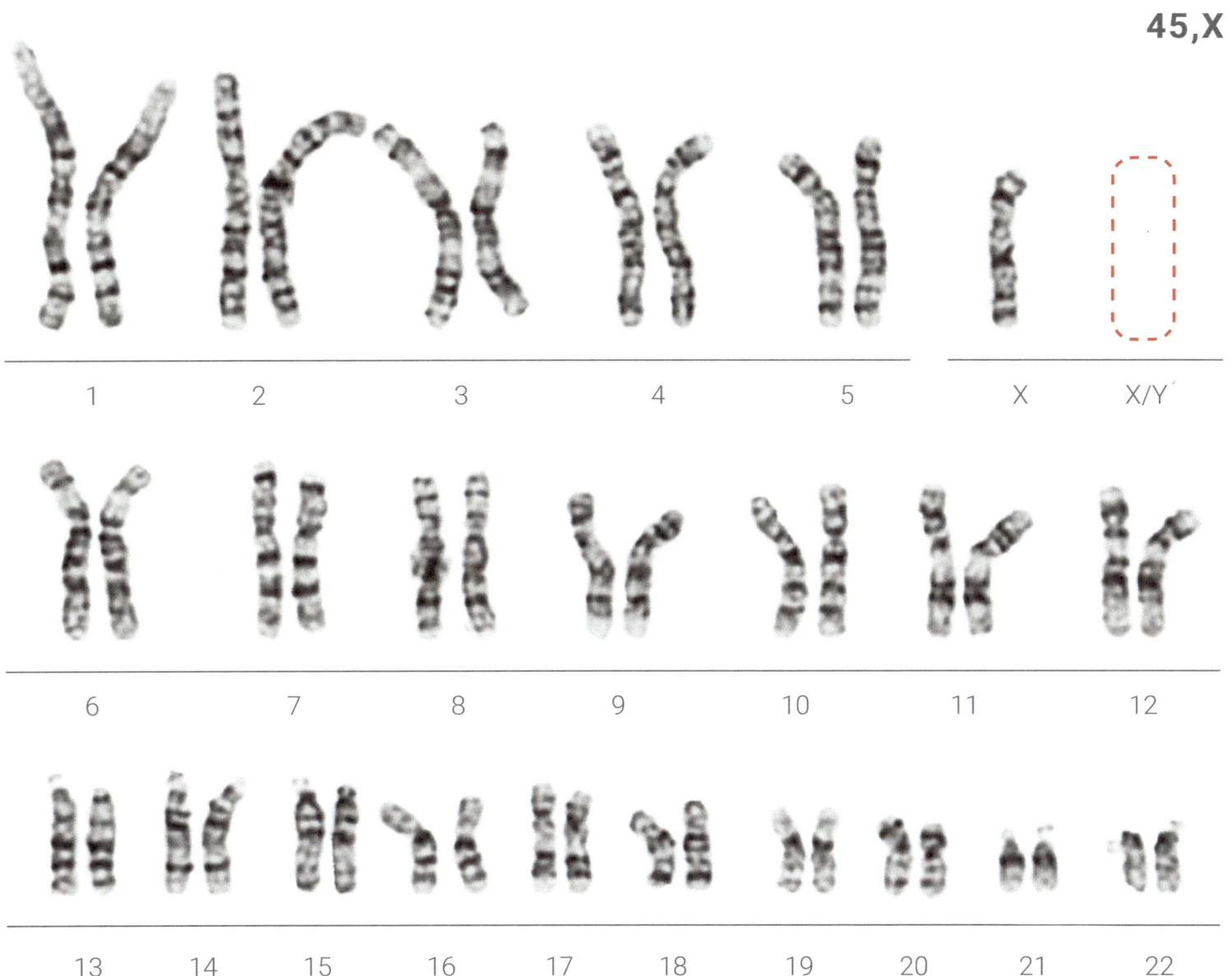

45,X

1 2 3 4 5 X X/Y

6 7 8 9 10 11 12

13 14 15 16 17 18 19 20 21 22

When part of an X-chromosome is missing = partial deletion Xp

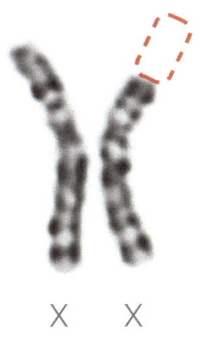
X X

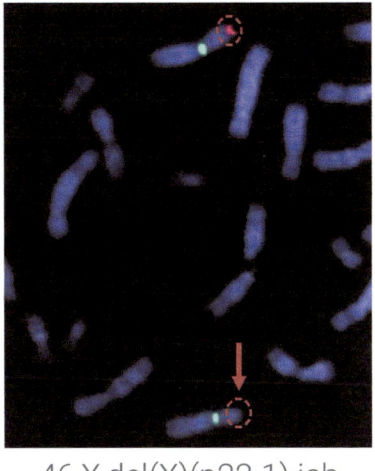

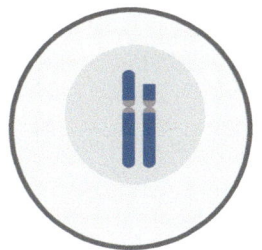
Somatic cell

46,X,del(X)(p22.1).ish

Ring chromosome X = 46,X,r(X)

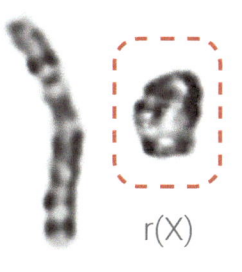
X

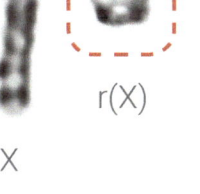
r(X)

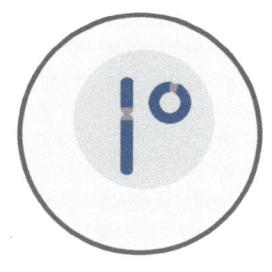
Somatic cell

Mosaic karyotype

45,X / 46,XX

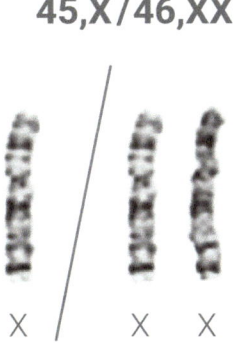
X / X X

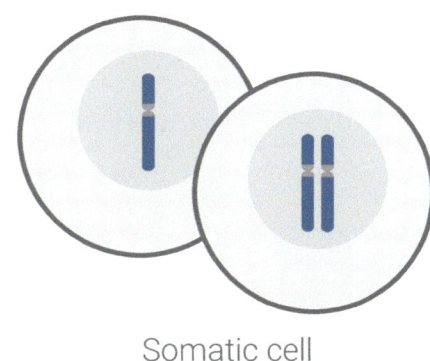
Somatic cell

45,X / 46,XY

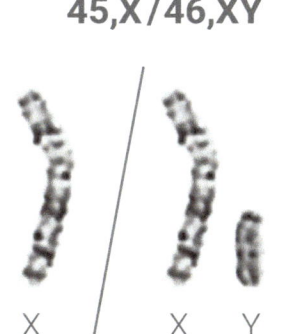
X / X Y

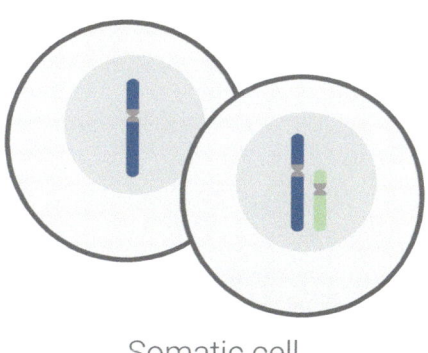
Somatic cell

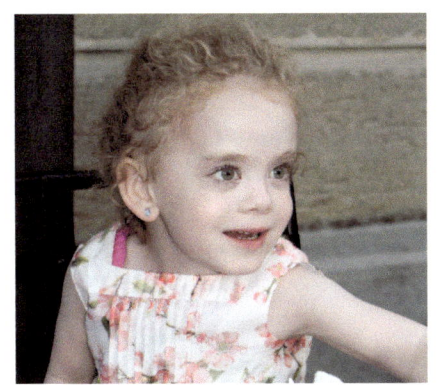

Girl (aged 4)
with Turner syndrome (45,X)

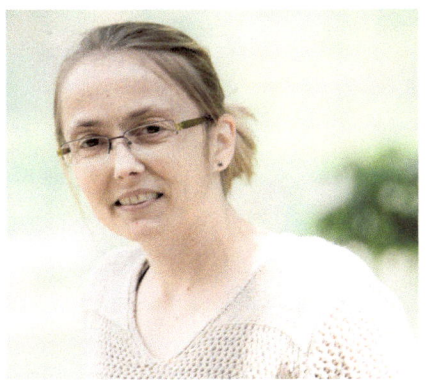

Woman (aged 42)
with Turner syndrome (45,X)

Incidence:

Approx. 1:2,000 live female births

A common cause of pregnancy loss

Prenatal ultrasound findings are often abnormal:

Increased nuchal translucency

Malformations, e.g. of the heart and kidneys

Short stature

Pterygium colli (webbed neck)

Heart defects

Kidney abnormalities

Delayed puberty

Streak gonads

No menstruation

Infertility

Swollen feet (infants)

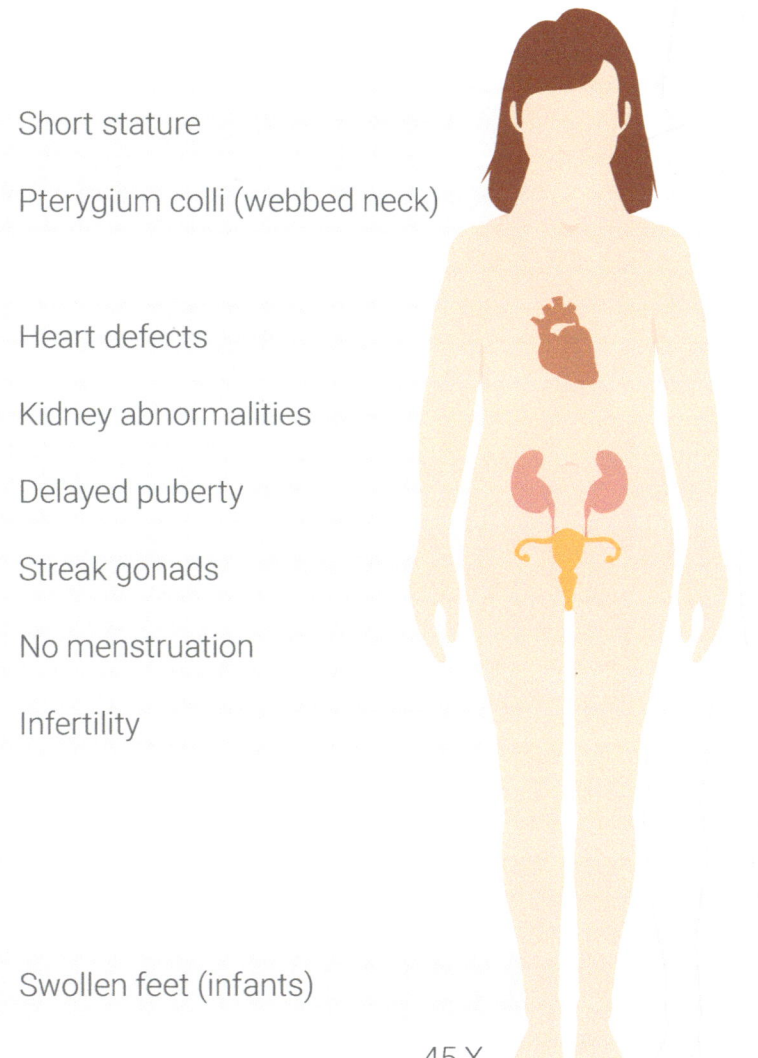

45,X   46,XX

47,XXX

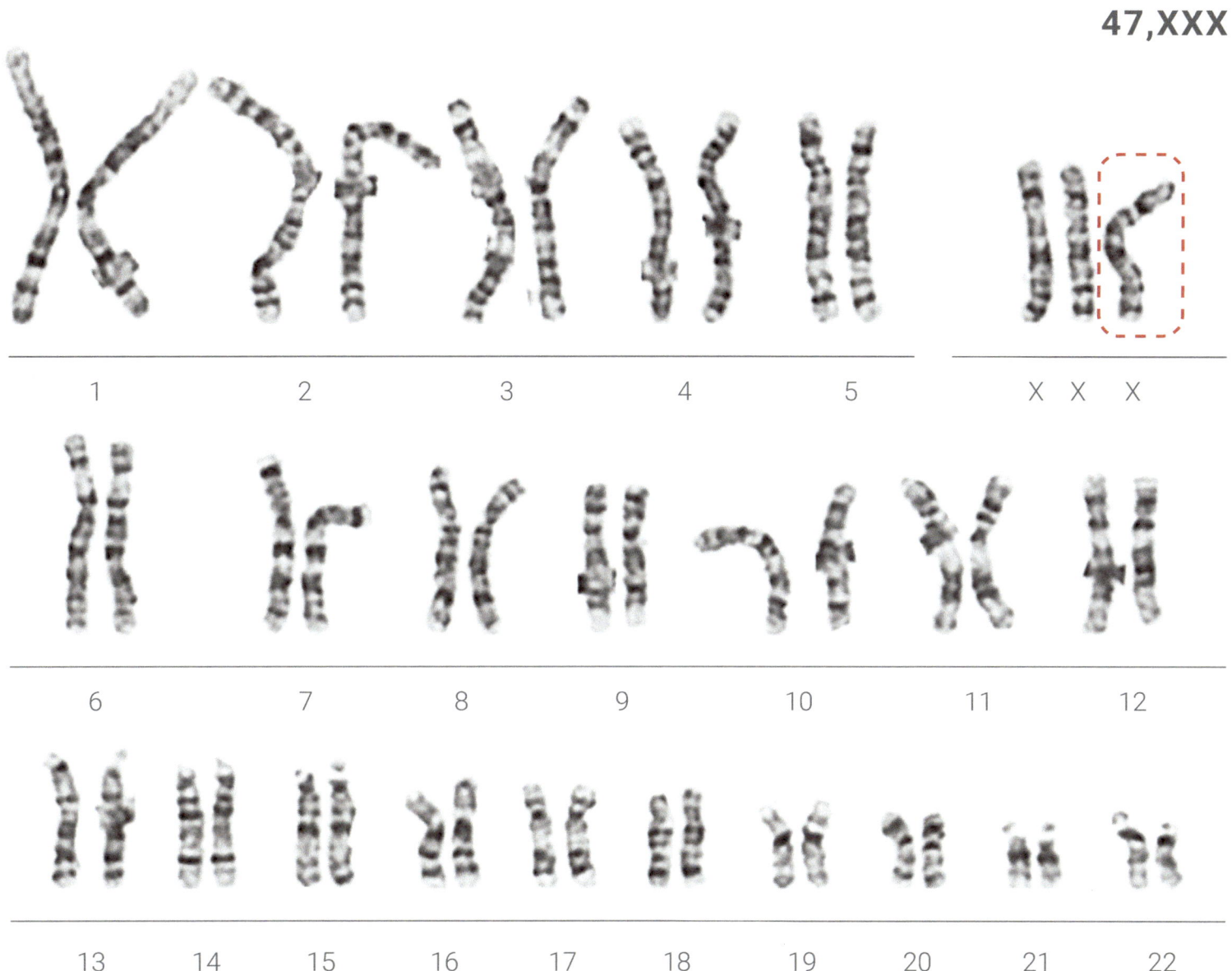

1 2 3 4 5 X X X

6 7 8 9 10 11 12

13 14 15 16 17 18 19 20 21 22

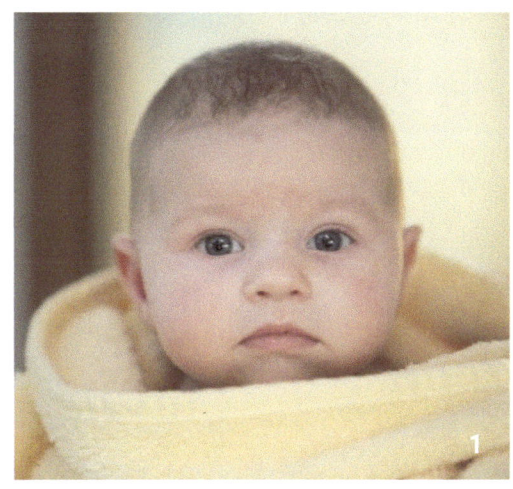 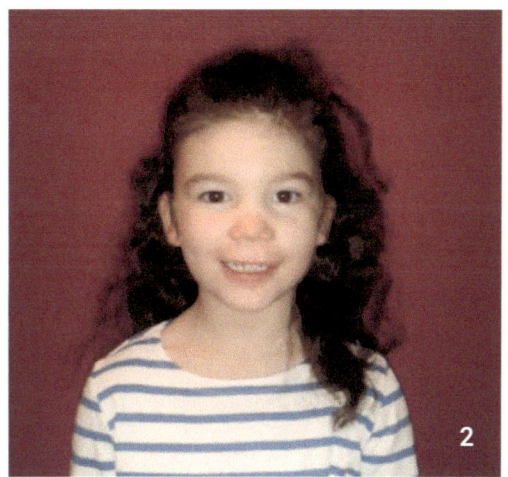 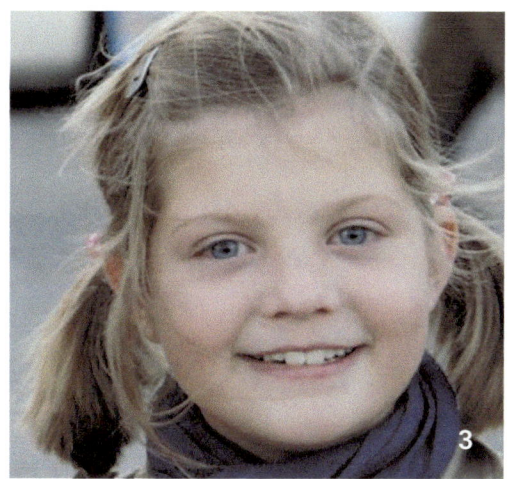

Girls with triple X syndrome (47,XXX) at the ages of 3 months (1), 5 years (2) and 8 years (3)

Incidence:

Approx. 1:1,000 girls/women

Therapy:

Psychomotor support, if necessary

Clinical features:

- Above-average height is common.
- Increased risk of mild developmental delay and learning difficulties.
- Increased risk of behavioural and emotional difficulties.
- Early menopause.

69,XXY

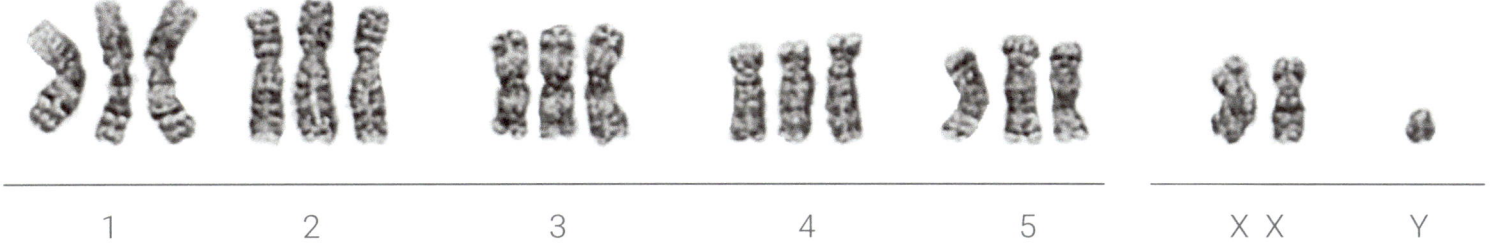

| 1 | 2 | 3 | 4 | 5 | X X | Y |

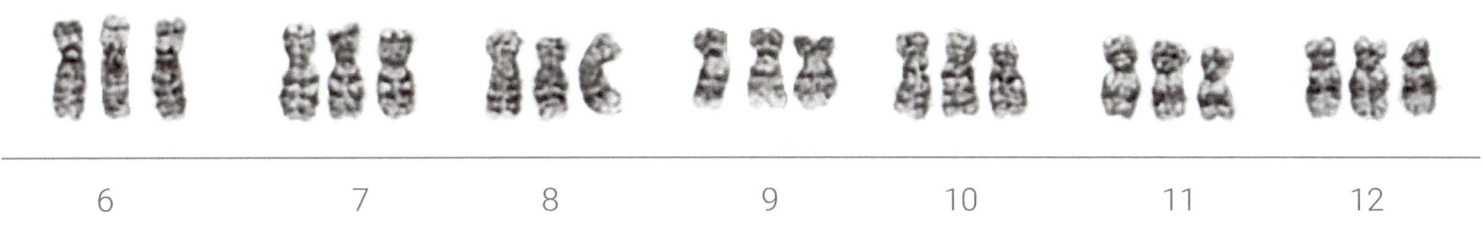

| 6 | 7 | 8 | 9 | 10 | 11 | 12 |

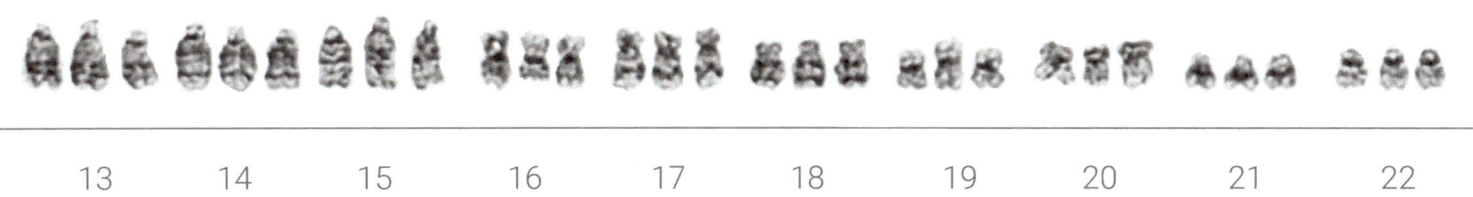

| 13 | 14 | 15 | 16 | 17 | 18 | 19 | 20 | 21 | 22 |

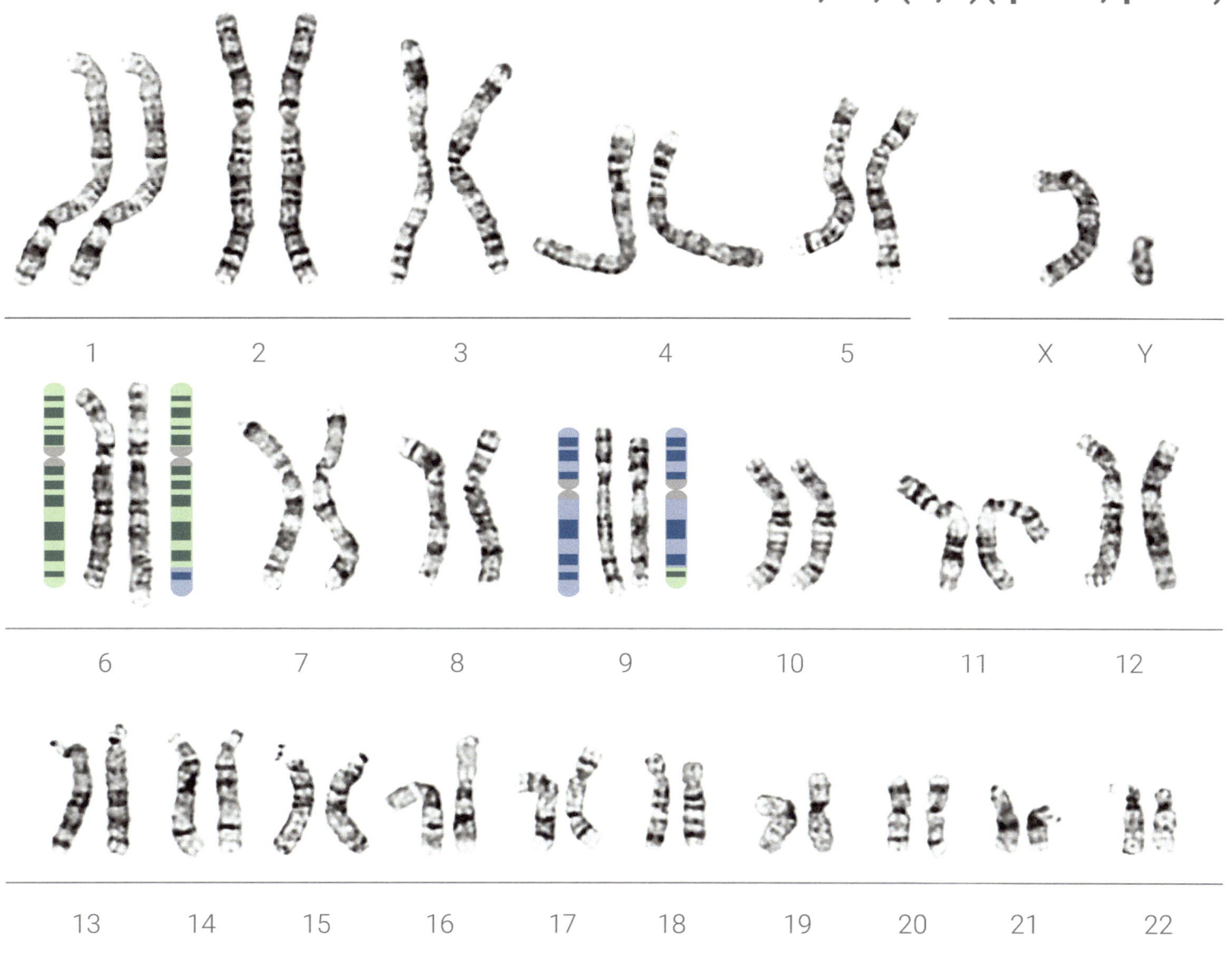

46,XY,t(6;9)(q25.3;q31.2)

1 2 3 4 5 X Y

6 7 8 9 10 11 12

13 14 15 16 17 18 19 20 21 22

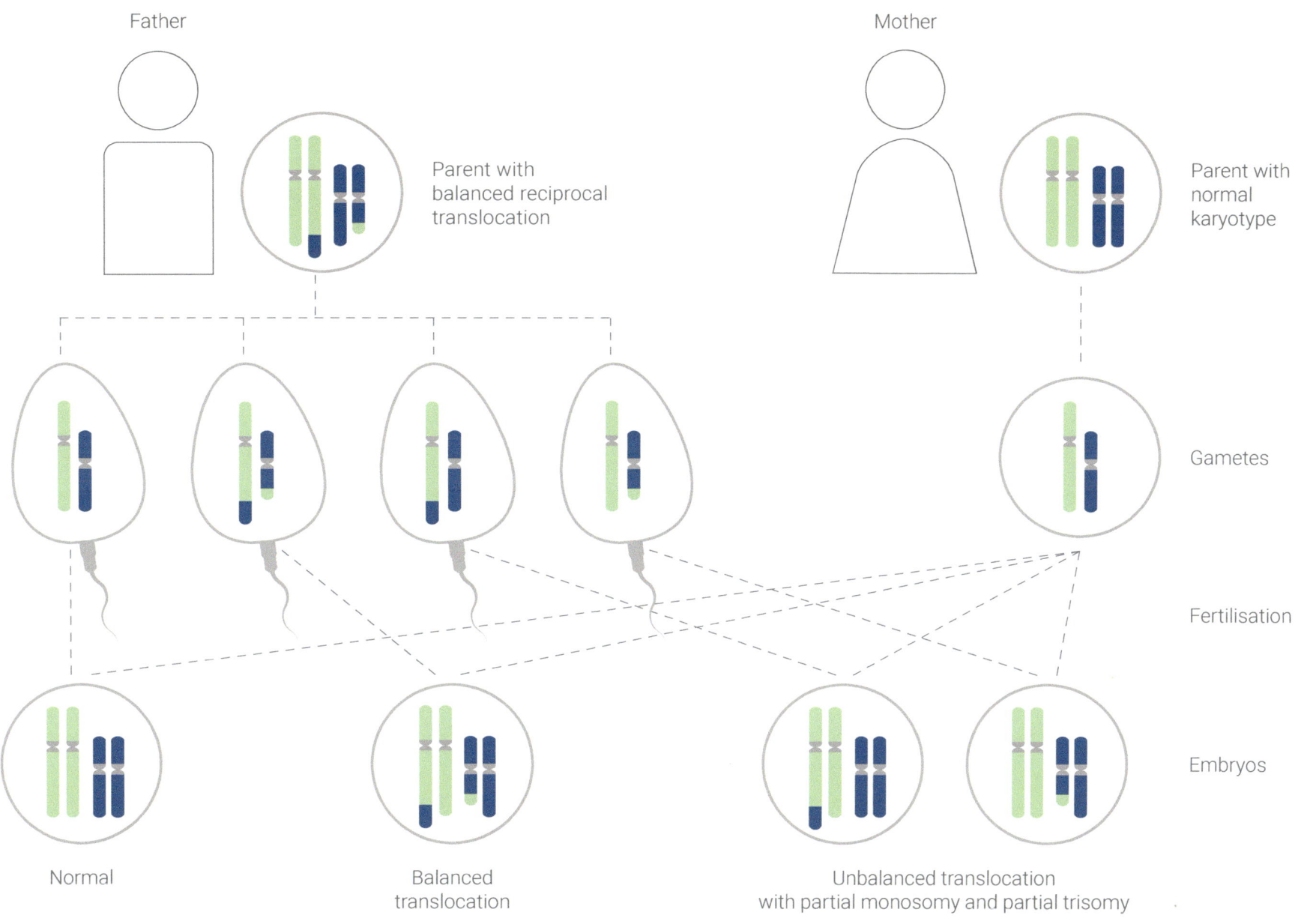

Father

Parent with balanced reciprocal translocation

Mother

Parent with normal karyotype

Gametes

Fertilisation

Embryos

Normal

Balanced translocation

Unbalanced translocation with partial monosomy and partial trisomy

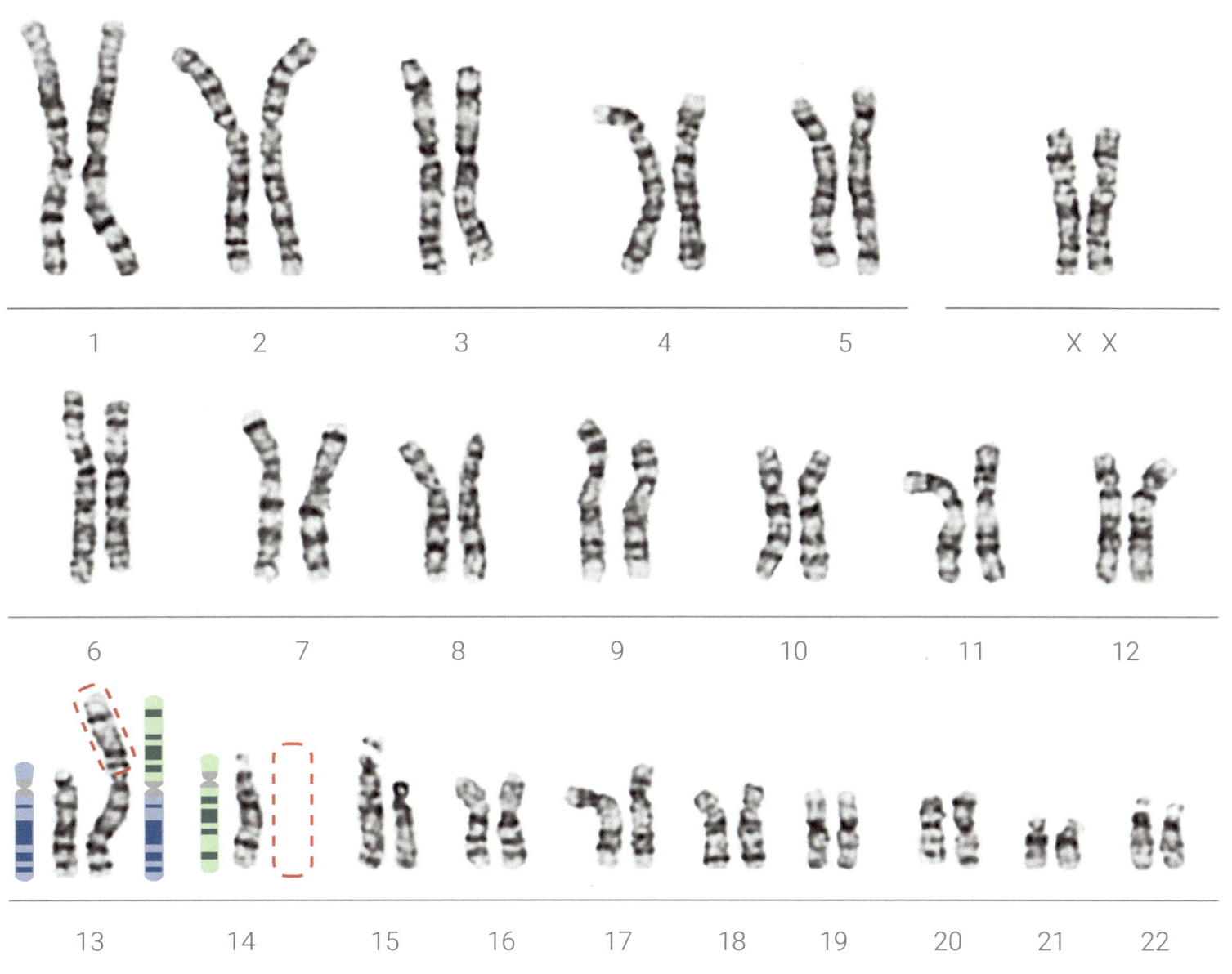

45,XX,der(13;14)(q10;q10)

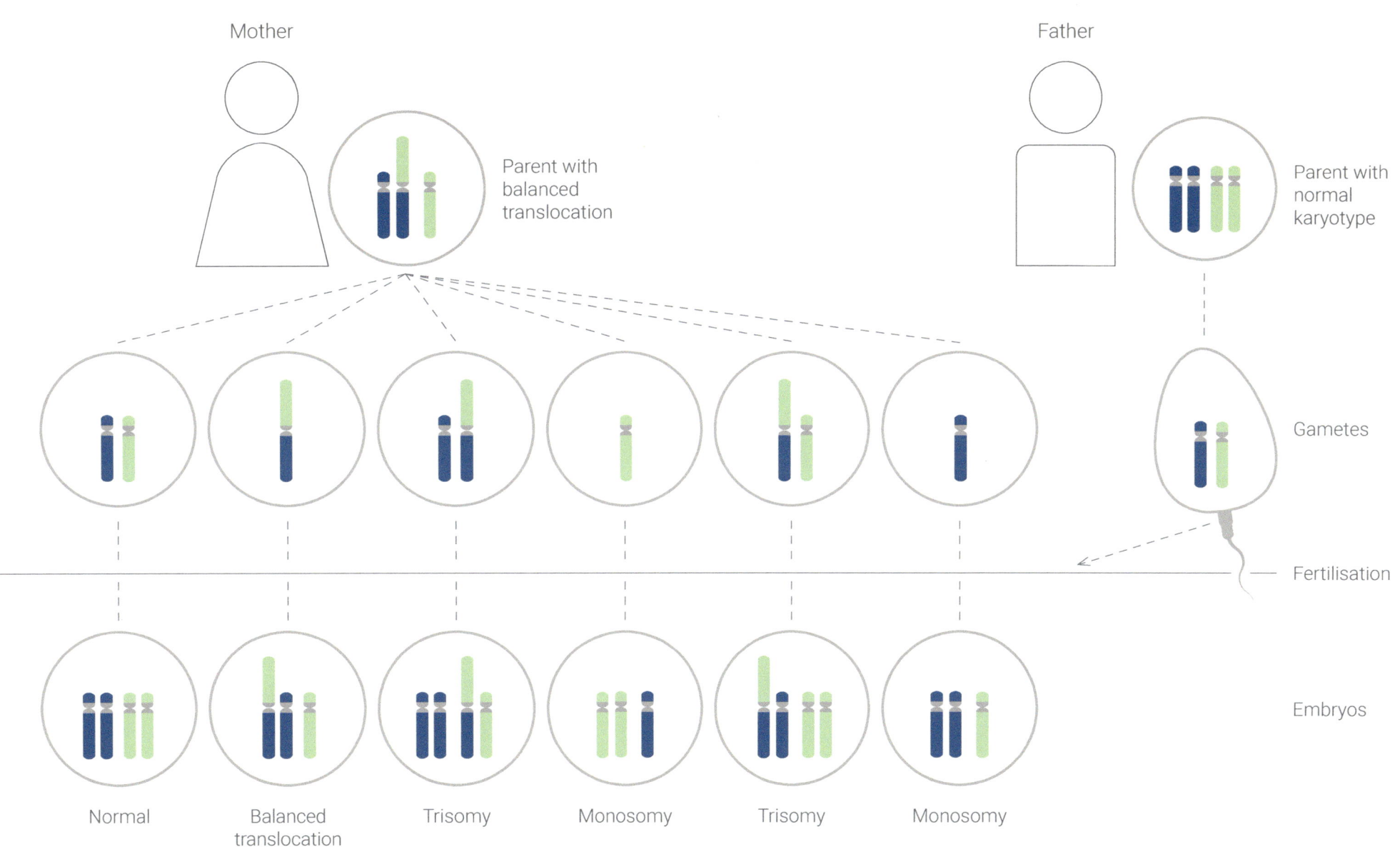

Mother

Father

Parent with balanced translocation

Parent with normal karyotype

Gametes

Fertilisation

Embryos

Normal

Balanced translocation

Trisomy

Monosomy

Trisomy

Monosomy

C Prenatal Diagnostics

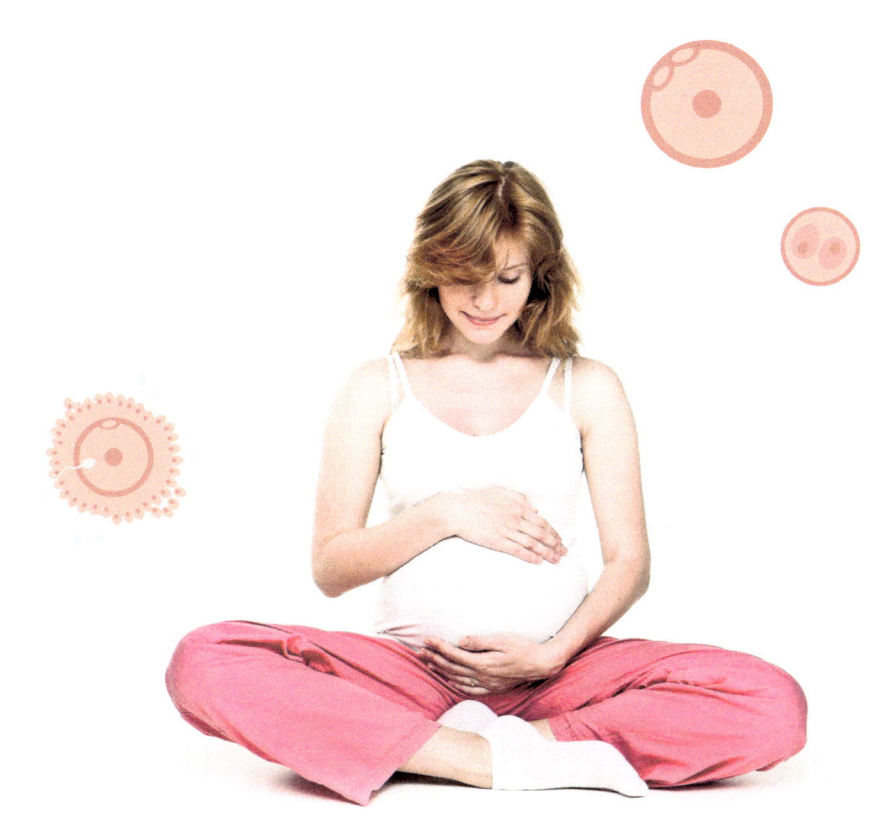

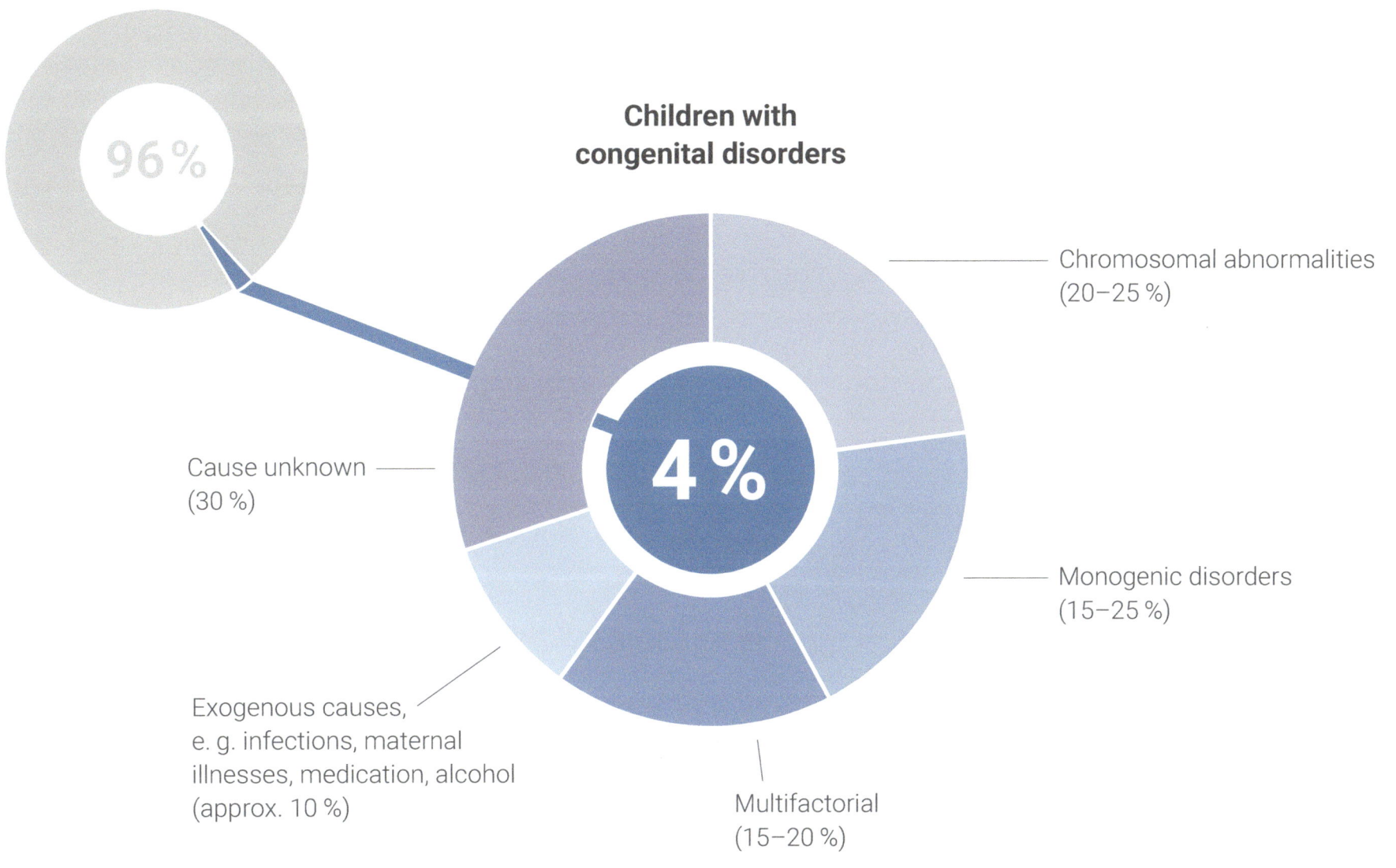

Healthy children

96 %

Children with
congenital disorders

4 %

Chromosomal abnormalities
(20–25 %)

Monogenic disorders
(15–25 %)

Multifactorial
(15–20 %)

Exogenous causes,
e. g. infections, maternal
illnesses, medication, alcohol
(approx. 10 %)

Cause unknown
(30 %)

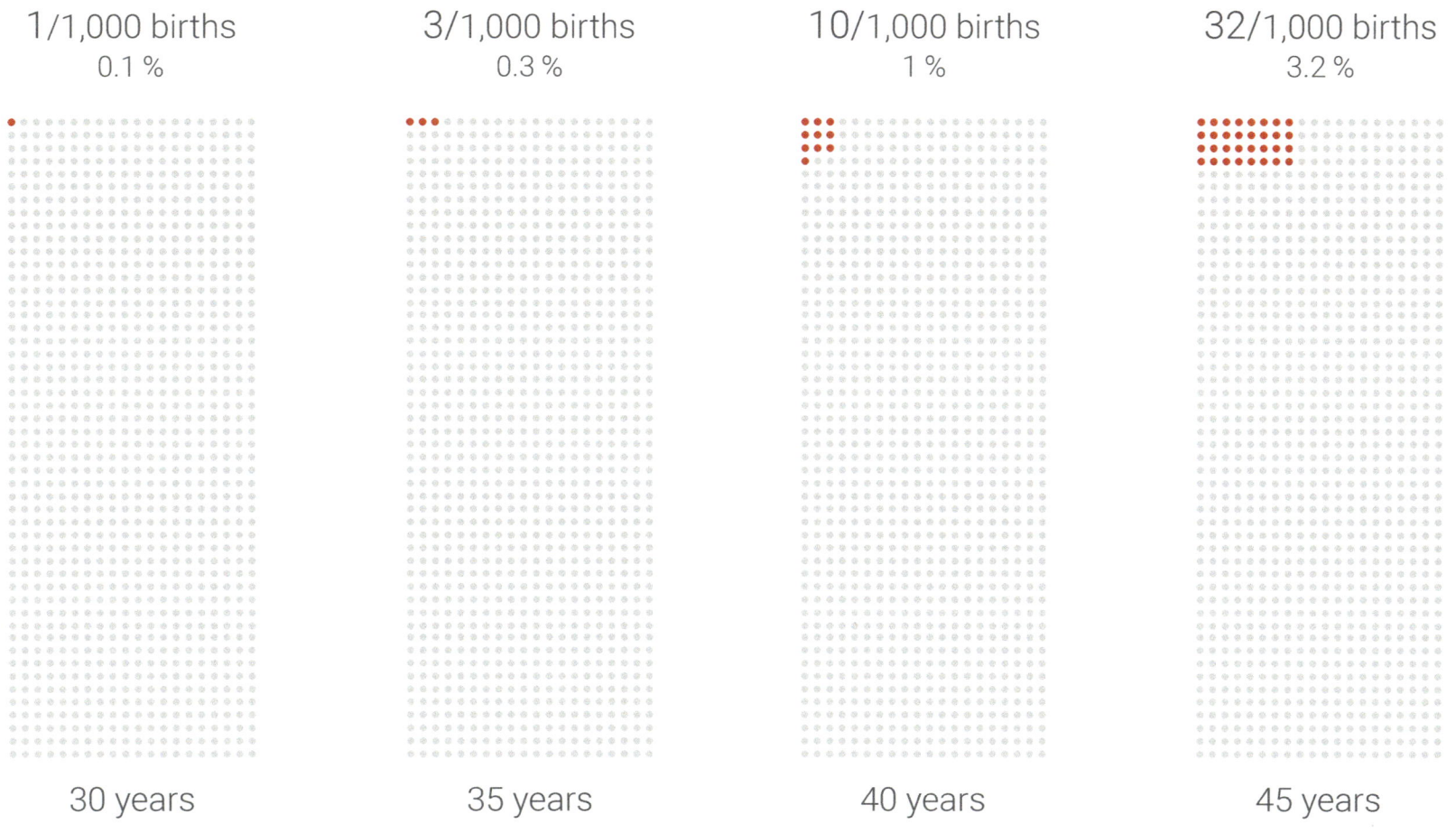

1/1,000 births
0.1 %

3/1,000 births
0.3 %

10/1,000 births
1 %

32/1,000 births
3.2 %

30 years

35 years

40 years

45 years

• Child with Down syndrome

	First Trimester[*]		Birth[**]	
Age	Trisomy 21	Total chromosomal abnormalities	Trisomy 21	Total chromosomal abnormalities
25	1 in 710	n.d.	1 in 4,000	1 in 1,000
30	1 in 470	n.d.	1 in 1,000	1 in 500
31	1 in 410	n.d.	1 in 850	1 in 450
32	1 in 350	n.d.	1 in 700	1 in 400
33	1 in 290	n.d.	1 in 600	1 in 330
34	1 in 235	n.d.	1 in 450	1 in 270
35	1 in 185	1 in 115	1 in 300	1 in 230
36	1 in 150	1 in 85	1 in 250	1 in 210
37	1 in 115	1 in 65	1 in 200	1 in 190
38	1 in 90	1 in 50	1 in 160	1 in 150
39	1 in 65	1 in 40	1 in 120	1 in 100
40	1 in 50	1 in 30	1 in 100	1 in 80
41	1 in 40	1 in 22	1 in 70	1 in 60
42	1 in 30	1 in 17	1 in 50	1 in 45
43	1 in 20	1 in 13	1 in 40	1 in 30
44	1 in 15	1 in 10	1 in 35	1 in 25

n.d. = no data available   * Snijders (1995), Hook (1992)   ** Morris (2002), Little (1995)

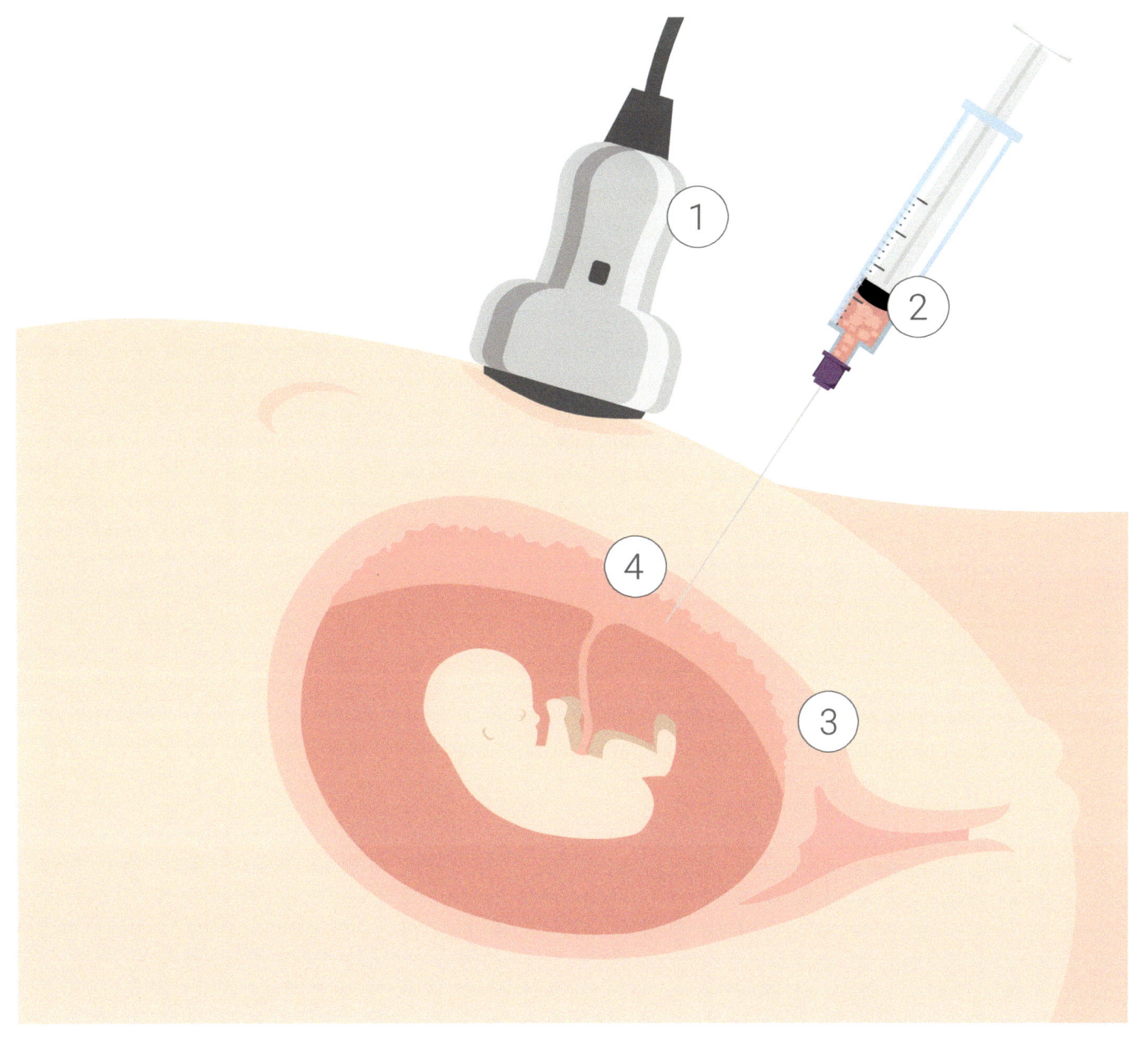

Chorionic villus sampling (CVS) = removal of a sample of tissue from the placenta

From the 11th week of pregnancy

Risk of miscarriage: 0.2–0.3 %

Results of chromosome analysis
Short-term culture: 1–2 days
Long-term culture: 10–14 days
DNA diagnosis possible

1 Ultrasound

2 Chorionic villus tissue

3 Uterus

4 Placenta

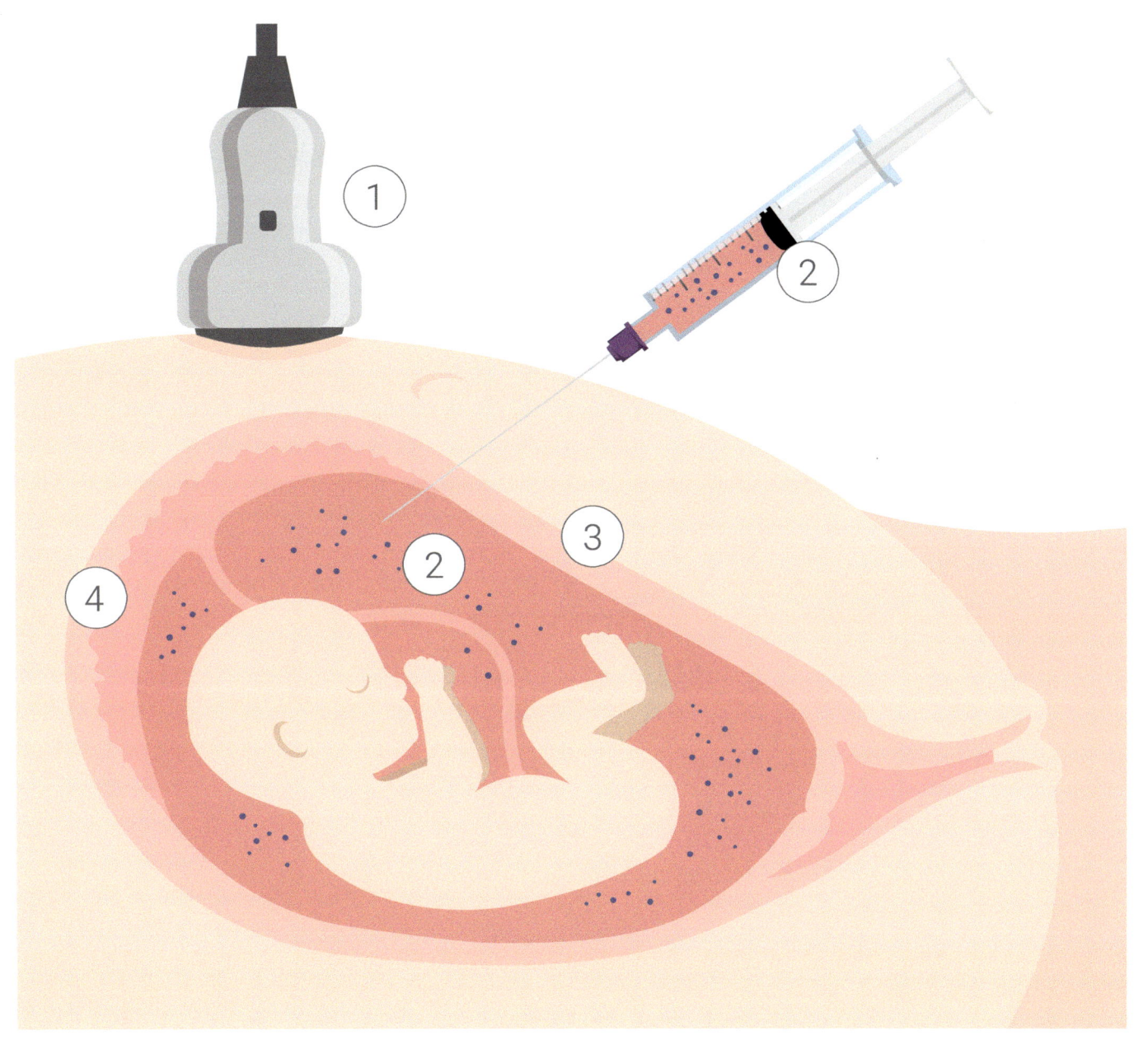

Amniocentesis (AC, "amnio") = amniotic fluid test

From the 15th/16th week of pregnancy

Risk of miscarriage: 0.1 %

Result of chromosome analysis
8–14 days
Rapid test available
DNA diagnosis possible

1. Ultrasound

2. Amniotic fluid containing foetal cells

3. Uterus

4. Placenta

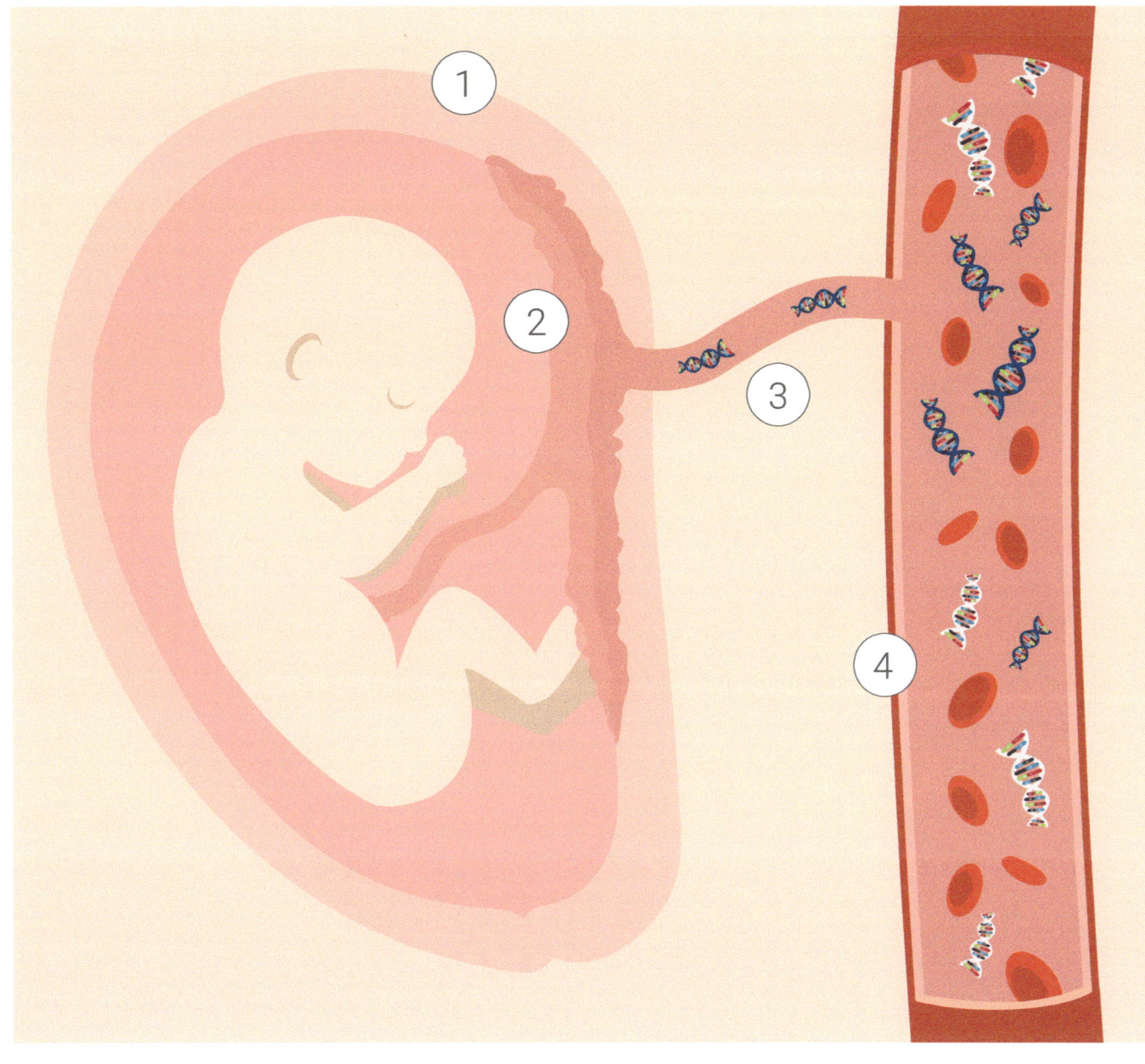

Non**i**nvasive **p**renatal **t**esting **(NIPT) =**

detection of foetal chromosome anomalies from the maternal blood

1) Uterus

2) Placenta

3) Foetal DNA

4) Maternal bloodstream (containing maternal and foetal DNA)

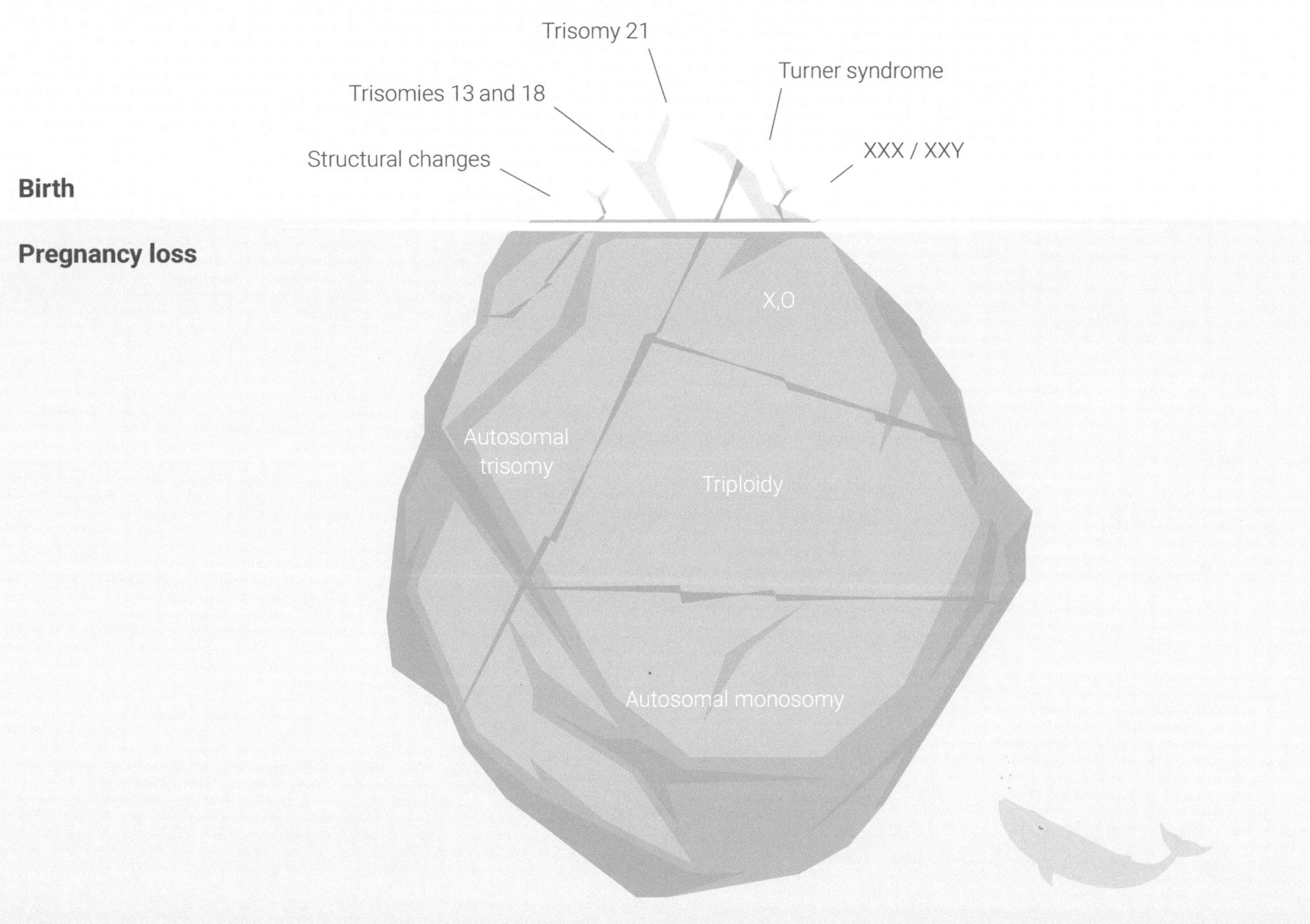

Birth

Pregnancy loss

Trisomy 21

Turner syndrome

Trisomies 13 and 18

XXX / XXY

Structural changes

X,O

Autosomal trisomy

Triploidy

Autosomal monosomy

D Inheritance Patterns

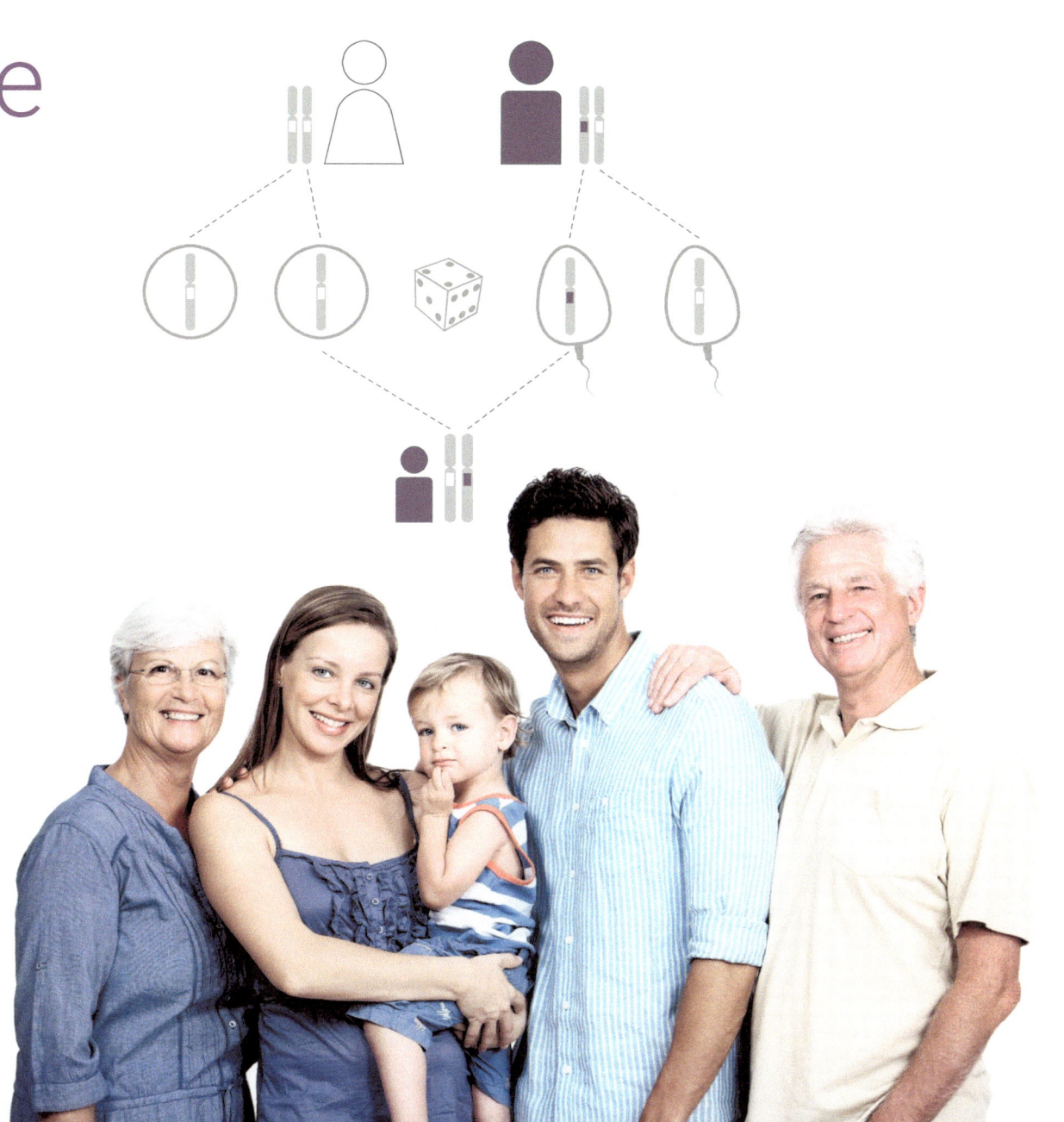

Autosomal dominant inheritance

Father: affected parent

Mother: healthy

Gametes

Fertilisation

Affected children: 50 %

Healthy children: 50 %

Characteristics:

- Affected individuals occur in successive generations.

- Women and men are equally affected.

- The inheritance risk for each child of an affected parent is 50 %.

Not affected

Affected

Autosomal recessive inheritance

Father: healthy carrier

Mother: healthy carrier

Not affected

Carrier

Affected

Gametes

Fertilisation

Characteristics:

- Both parents are carriers:
  25 % risk of an affected child.

- Girls and boys are equally affected.

- Affected individuals commonly occur
  in one generation only.

- There is an increased risk of affected
  offspring in consanguineous marriages.

Affected children:
25 %

Carriers:
50 %

Non-carriers:
25 %

Healthy children:
75 %

X-linked inheritance

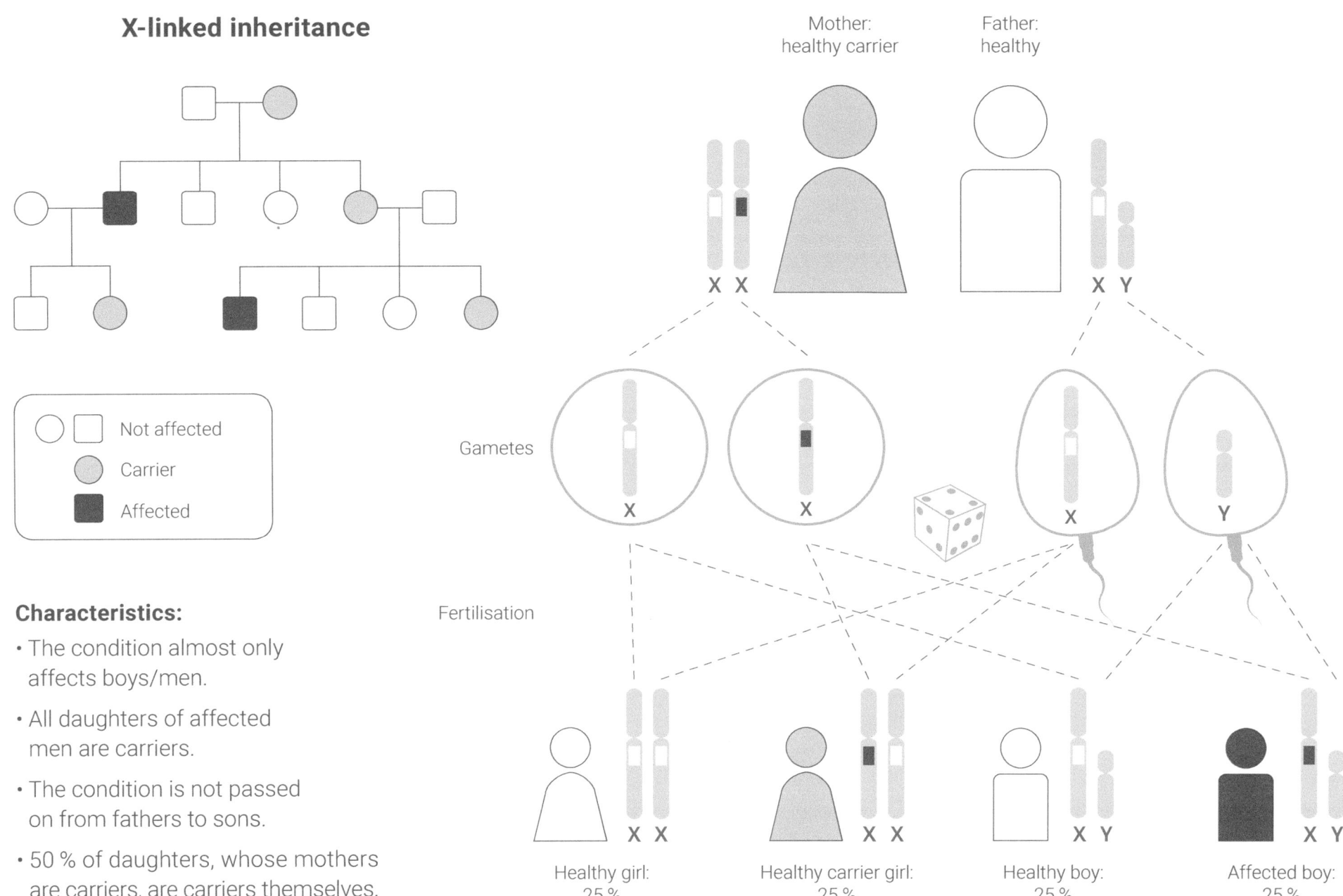

Mother:
healthy carrier

Father:
healthy

X X

X Y

Gametes

X

X

X

Y

Fertilisation

Healthy girl:
25 %

X X

Healthy carrier girl:
25 %

X X

Healthy boy:
25 %

X Y

Affected boy:
25 %

X Y

Not affected

Carrier

Affected

Characteristics:

• The condition almost only
  affects boys/men.

• All daughters of affected
  men are carriers.

• The condition is not passed
  on from fathers to sons.

• 50 % of daughters, whose mothers
  are carriers, are carriers themselves.

Mitochondrial inheritance

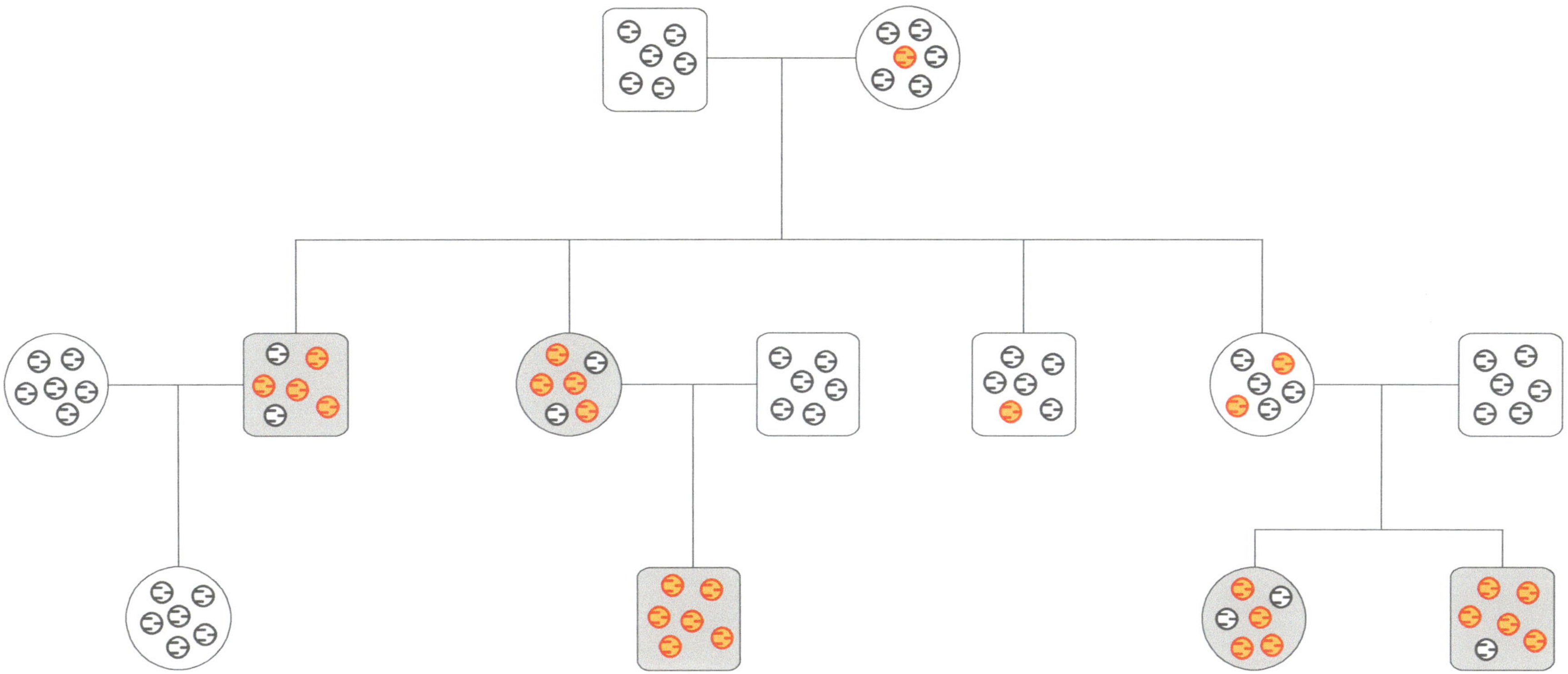

Characteristics:

- Mitochondria are inherited from the mother only: all offspring may be affected.
- Mitochondrial disease becomes apparent when the number of mutated mitochondria in the cell exceeds a threshold level.
- Sons/men cannot transmit the predisposition/disorder.

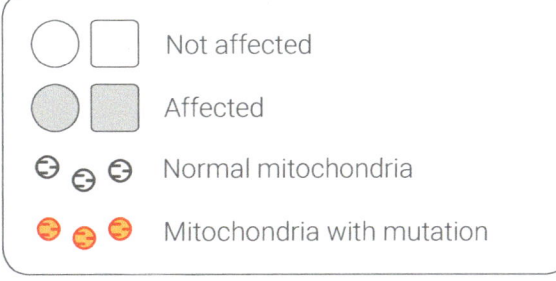

Not affected

Affected

Normal mitochondria

Mitochondria with mutation

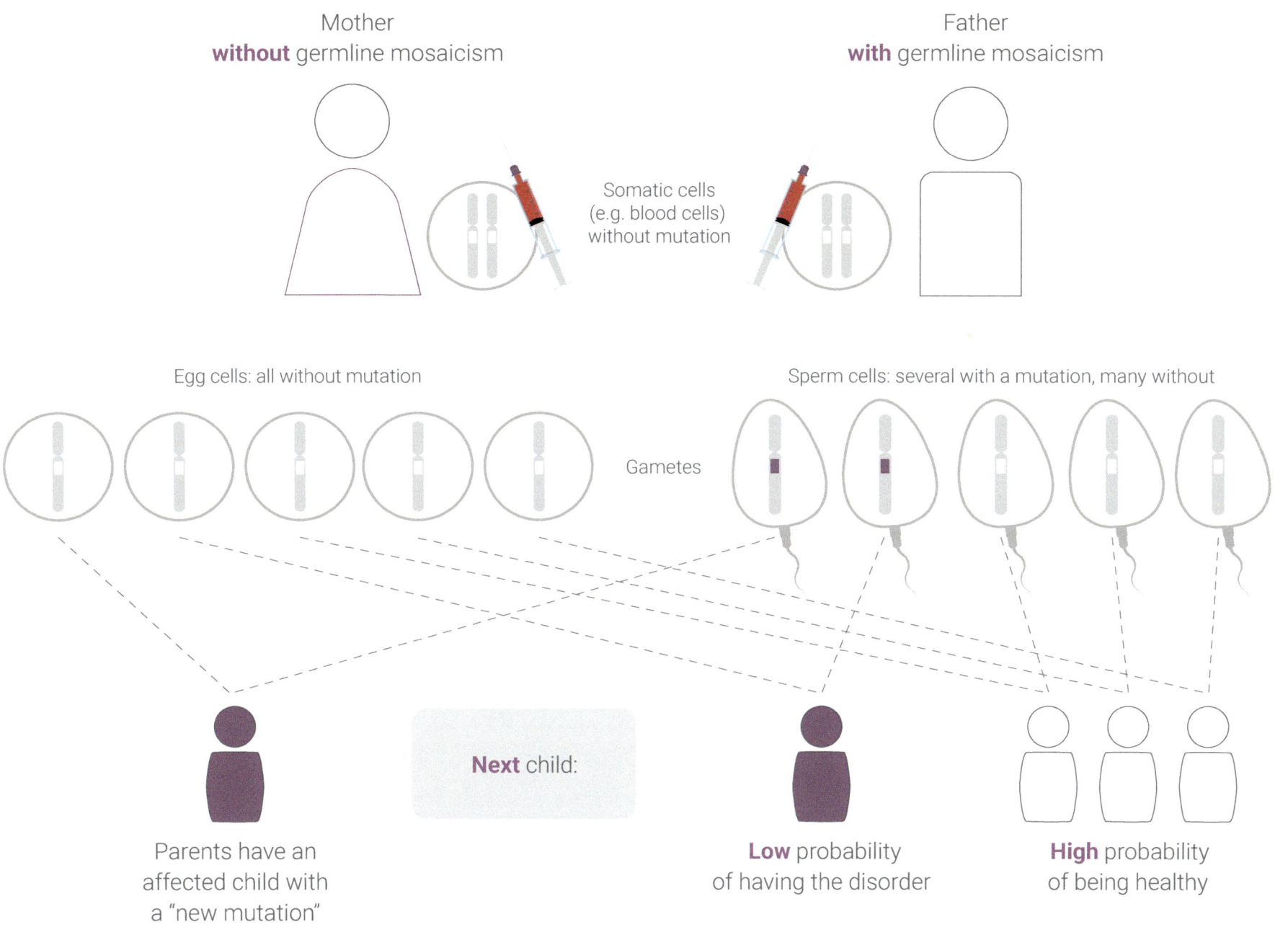

Mother
without germline mosaicism

Father
with germline mosaicism

Somatic cells
(e.g. blood cells)
without mutation

Egg cells: all without mutation

Sperm cells: several with a mutation, many without

Gametes

Next child:

Parents have an
affected child with
a "new mutation"

Low probability
of having the disorder

High probability
of being healthy

E Reproduction

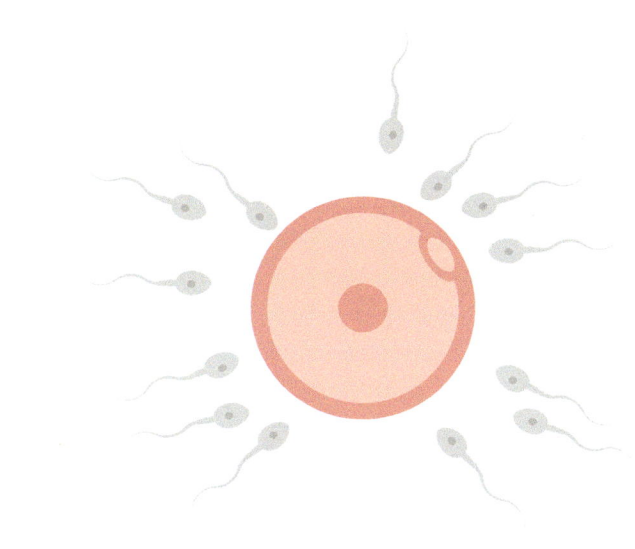

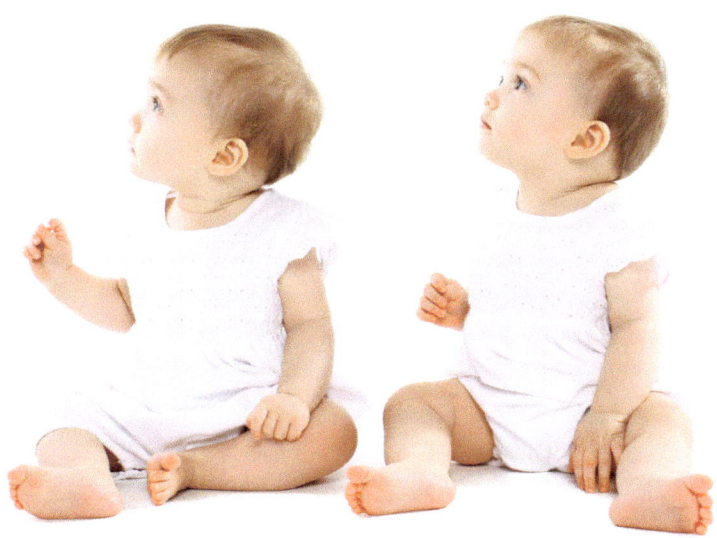

**One in six pregnancies
ends in miscarriage**

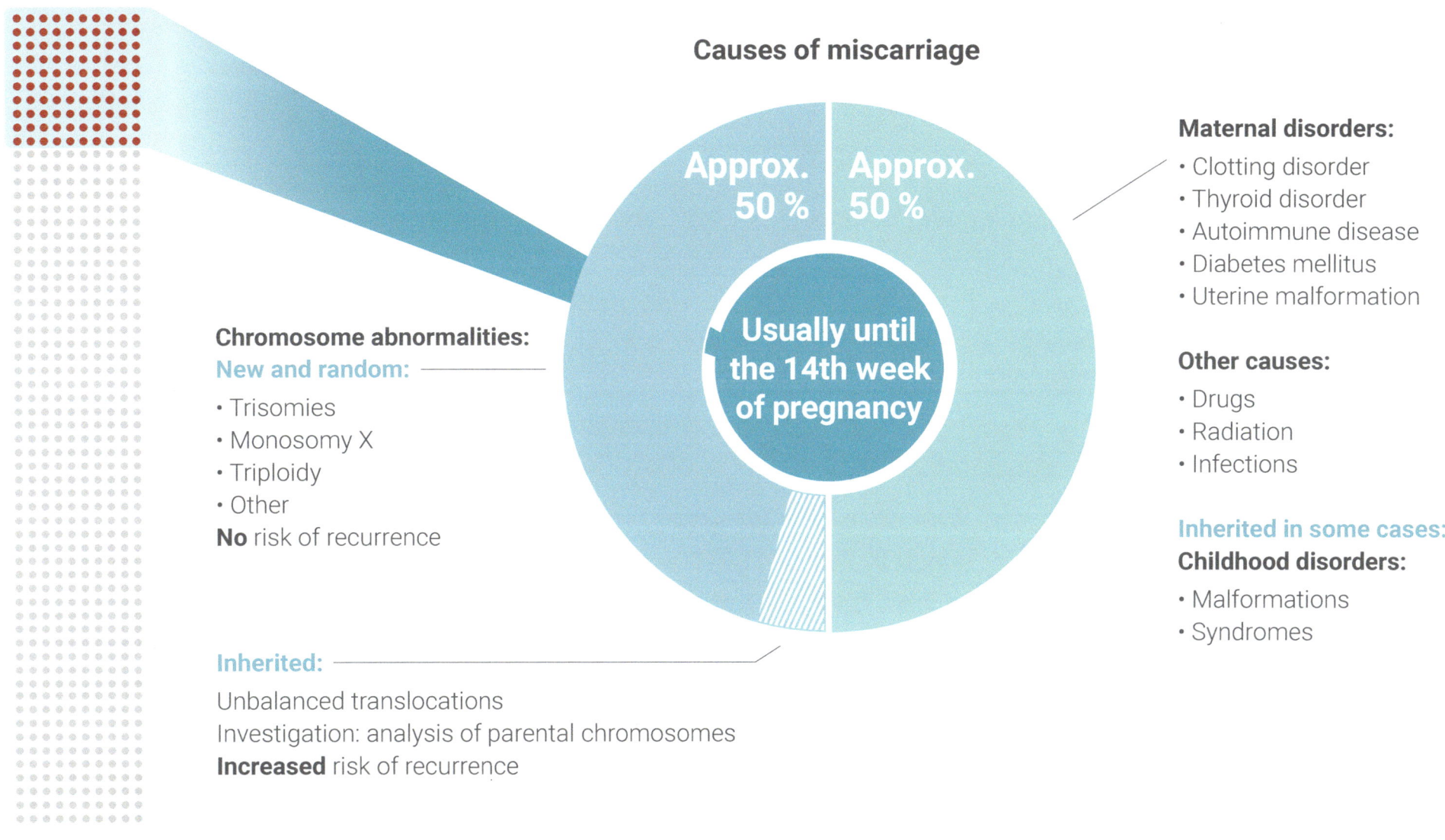

Causes of miscarriage

Approx. 50 %

Approx. 50 %

Usually until the 14th week of pregnancy

Chromosome abnormalities:

New and random:

• Trisomies
• Monosomy X
• Triploidy
• Other
No risk of recurrence

Inherited:

Unbalanced translocations
Investigation: analysis of parental chromosomes
Increased risk of recurrence

Maternal disorders:

• Clotting disorder
• Thyroid disorder
• Autoimmune disease
• Diabetes mellitus
• Uterine malformation

Other causes:

• Drugs
• Radiation
• Infections

Inherited in some cases:
Childhood disorders:

• Malformations
• Syndromes

600 pregnancies

Balanced Robertsonian translocation t(13;14)
in the case of a healthy mother

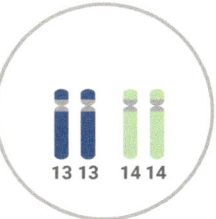

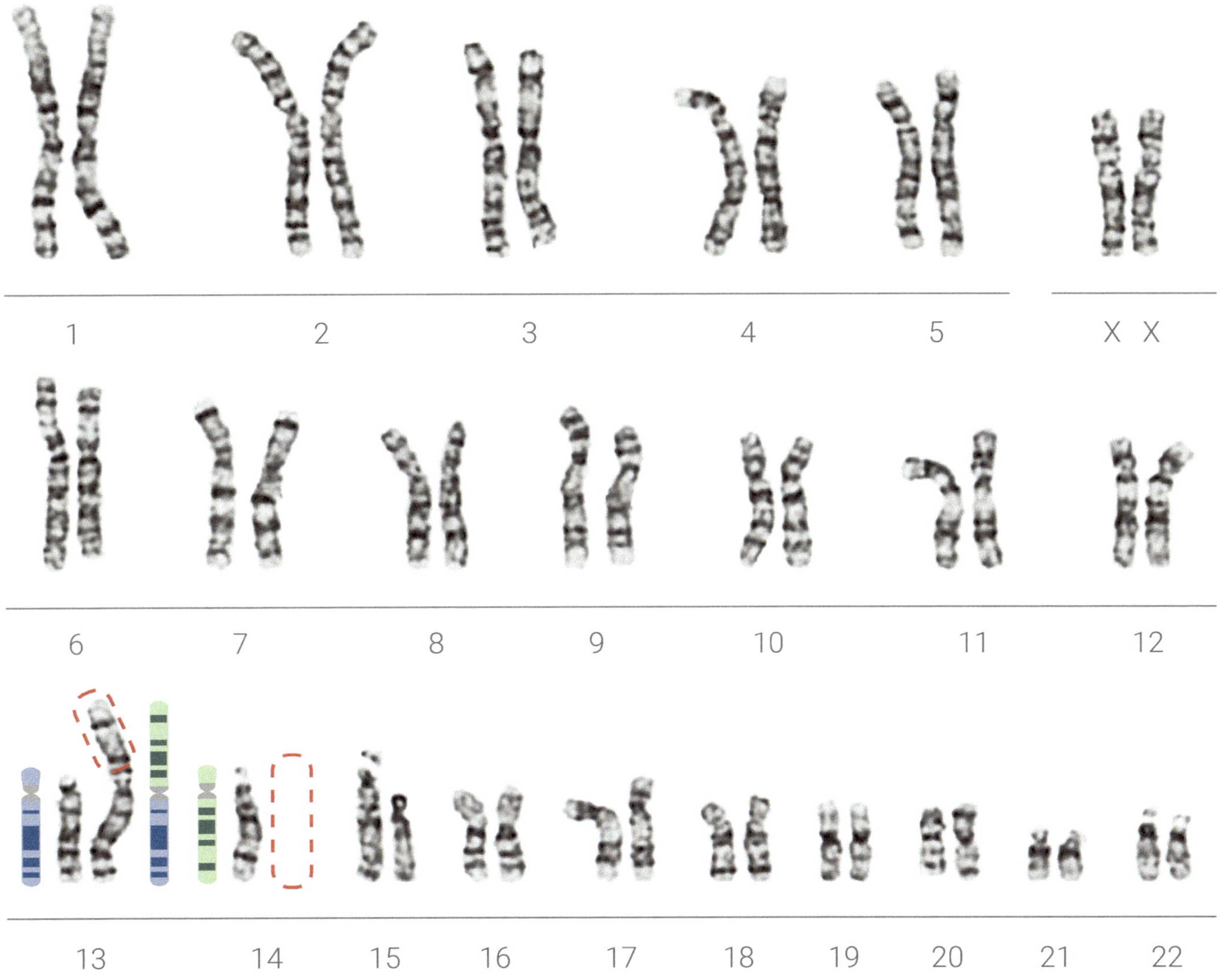

Normal

Healthy children

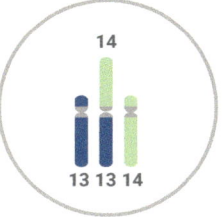

Balanced translocation

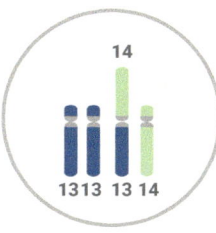

Trisomy 13

Miscarriage is the most common outcome

Birth of a child with severe physical and intellectual disabilities is rare

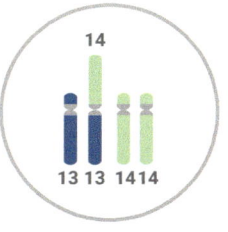

Trisomy 14

Miscarriage

1   2   3   4   5   X X

6   7   8   9   10   11   12

13   14   15   16   17   18   19   20   21   22

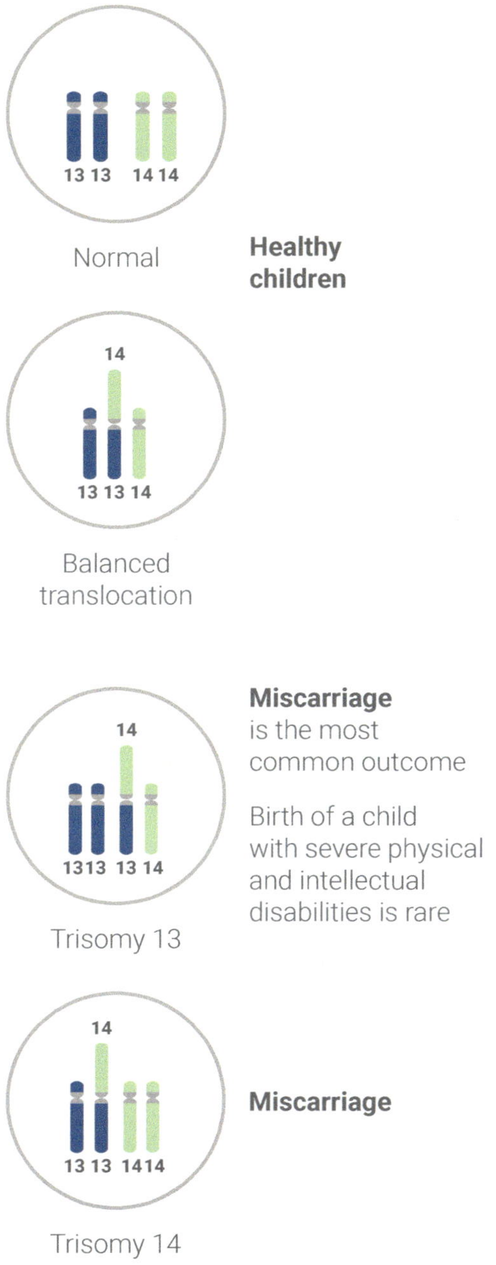

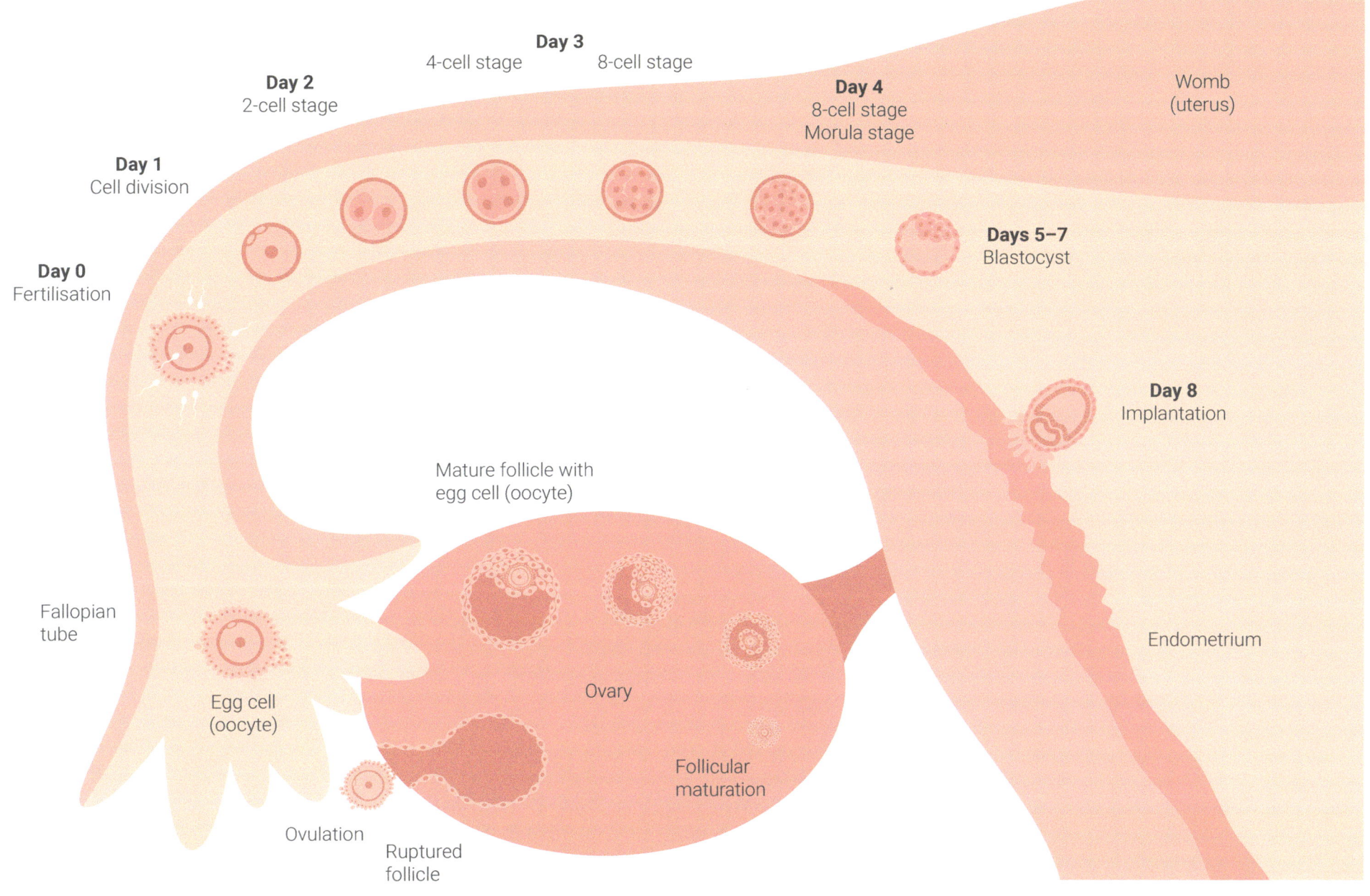

Day 3
4-cell stage   8-cell stage

Day 2
2-cell stage

Day 4
8-cell stage
Morula stage

Womb
(uterus)

Day 1
Cell division

Days 5–7
Blastocyst

Day 0
Fertilisation

Day 8
Implantation

Mature follicle with
egg cell (oocyte)

Fallopian
tube

Endometrium

Egg cell
(oocyte)

Ovary

Follicular
maturation

Ovulation

Ruptured
follicle

Woman: Hormone treatment and egg retrieval

Male: Sperm sample or testicular biopsy (if there is azoospermia)

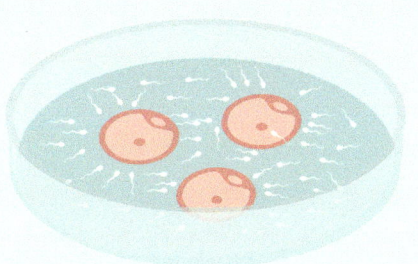

Egg cells
are fertilised
by sperm cells

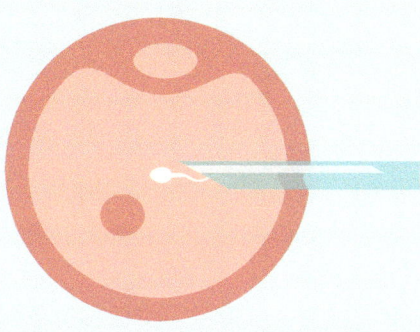

One sperm cell
is injected into
the egg cell

IVF = in vitro fertilisation

**ICSI = intracytoplasmic
sperm injection**

Woman: Embryos are transferred to the uterus

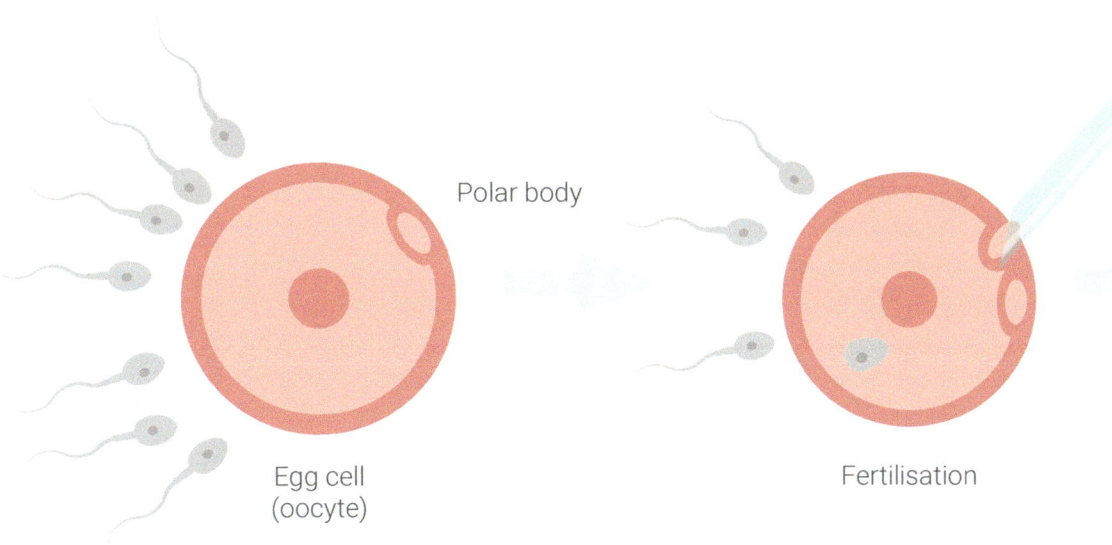

Polar body

Egg cell
(oocyte)

Fertilisation

PBD = polar body diagnosis
to screen for maternally
inherited disorders

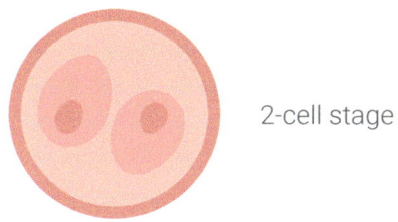

2-cell stage

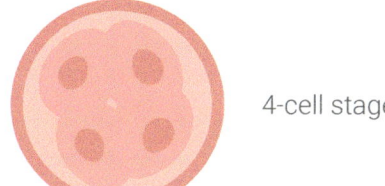

4-cell stage

PID = preimplantation diagnosis
to screen for maternally and
paternally inherited disorders

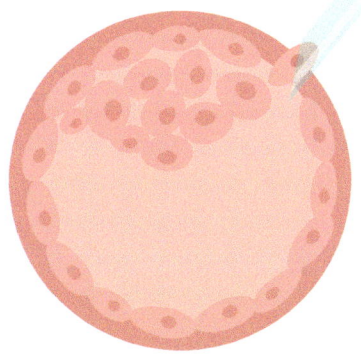

Blastocyst (day 5)

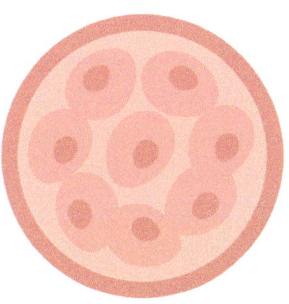

8-cell stage

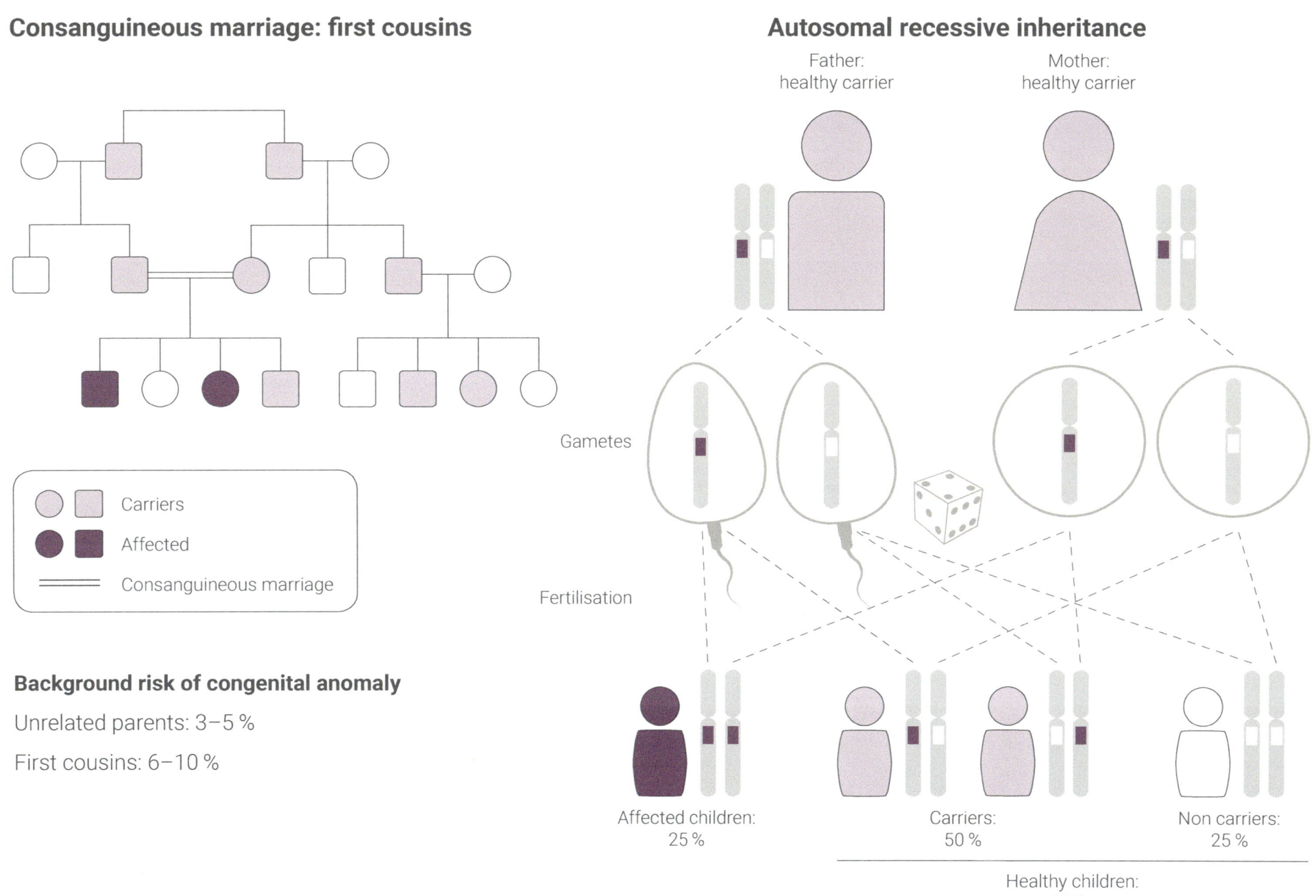

Consanguineous marriage: first cousins

Carriers
Affected
Consanguineous marriage

Background risk of congenital anomaly

Unrelated parents: 3–5 %

First cousins: 6–10 %

Autosomal recessive inheritance

Father:
healthy carrier

Mother:
healthy carrier

Gametes

Fertilisation

Affected children:
25 %

Carriers:
50 %

Non carriers:
25 %

Healthy children:
75 %

F Cancer

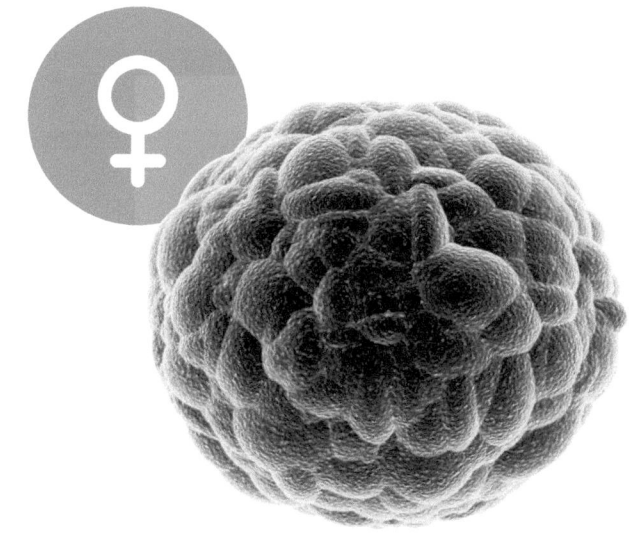

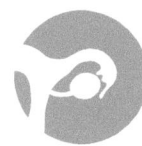

Sporadic cancer

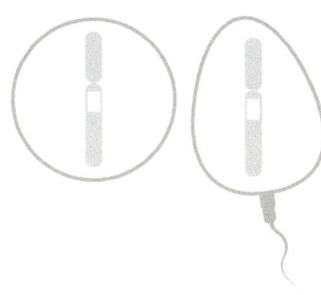

Two successive random mutations in both alleles of a tumour suppressor gene in a somatic cell

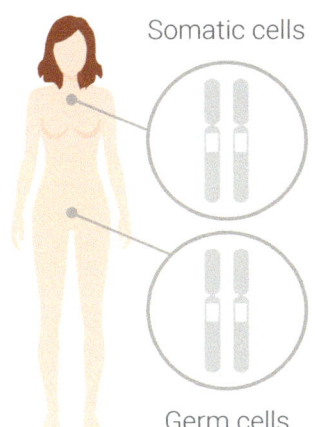

Somatic cells

Germ cells

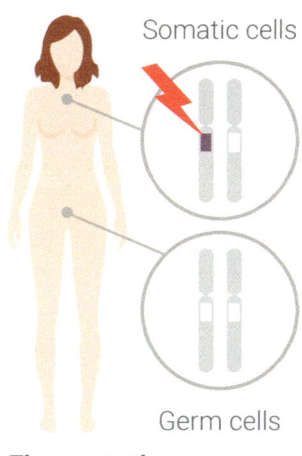

Somatic cells

Germ cells

First mutation

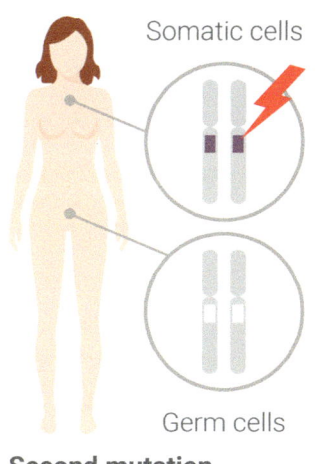

Somatic cells

Germ cells

Second mutation

Next Generation

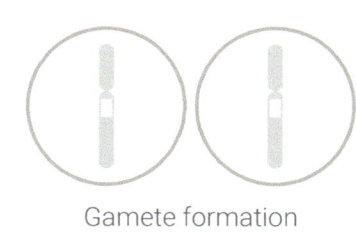

Gamete formation

Inherited cancer

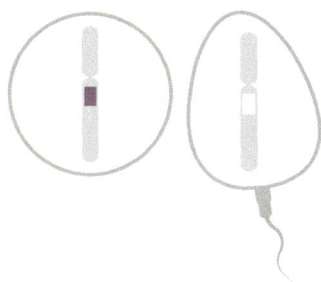

Germline mutation in a tumour suppressor gene and a second random mutation in the other allele

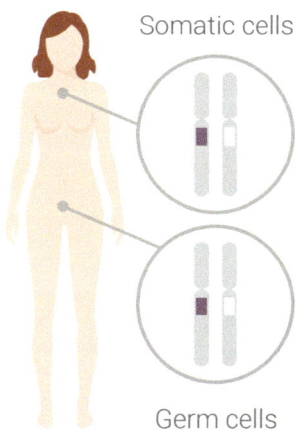

Somatic cells

Germ cells

First mutation congenitally present in all somatic and germ cells

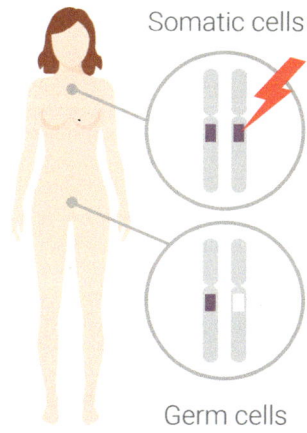

Somatic cells

Germ cells

Second mutation in a somatic cell

Next Generation

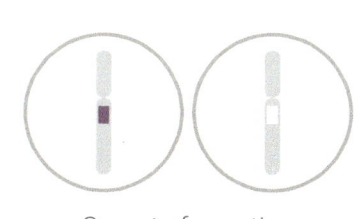

Gamete formation

Sporadic cancer

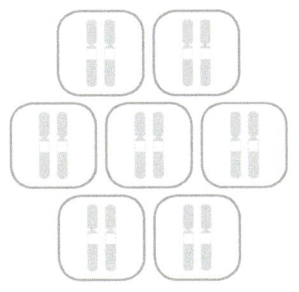

Normal
cell growth

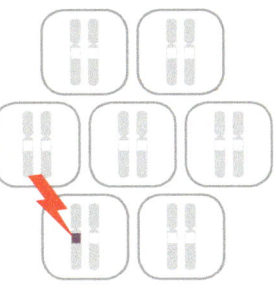

First mutation

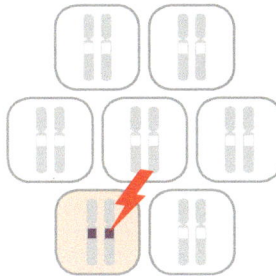

Second mutation

Inherited cancer

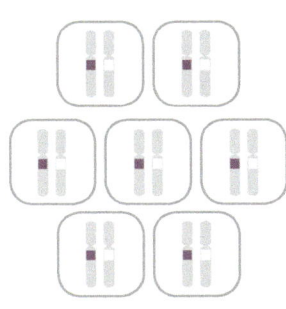

First mutation
contained in all cells

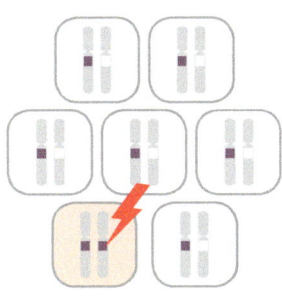

Second mutation

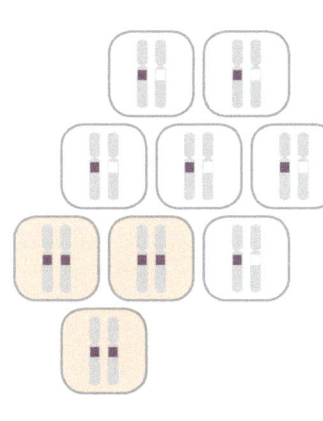

Tumour cells grow faster
than normal cells

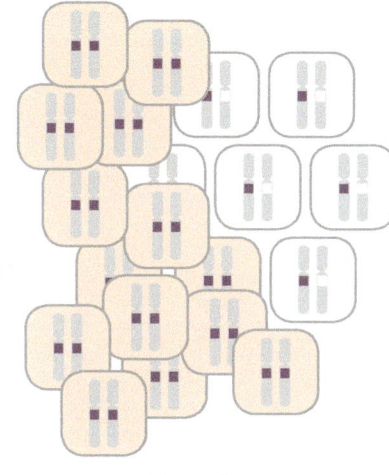

Complete
tumour

Development of bowel cancer
Cascade of different gene mutations

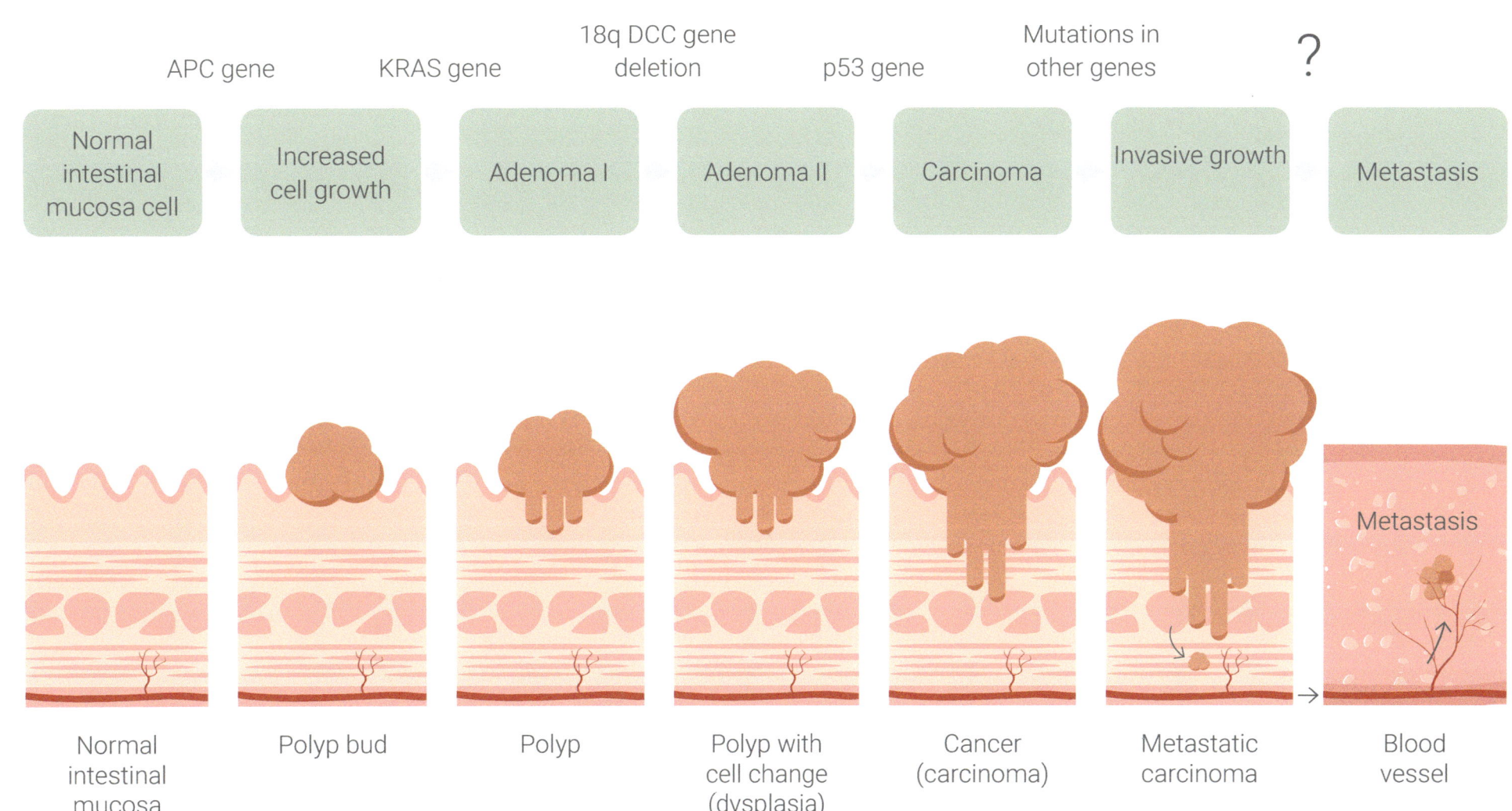

APC gene · KRAS gene · 18q DCC gene deletion · p53 gene · Mutations in other genes · ?

Normal intestinal mucosa cell → Increased cell growth → Adenoma I → Adenoma II → Carcinoma → Invasive growth → Metastasis

Normal intestinal mucosa · Polyp bud · Polyp · Polyp with cell change (dysplasia) · Cancer (carcinoma) · Metastatic carcinoma · Blood vessel

Metastasis

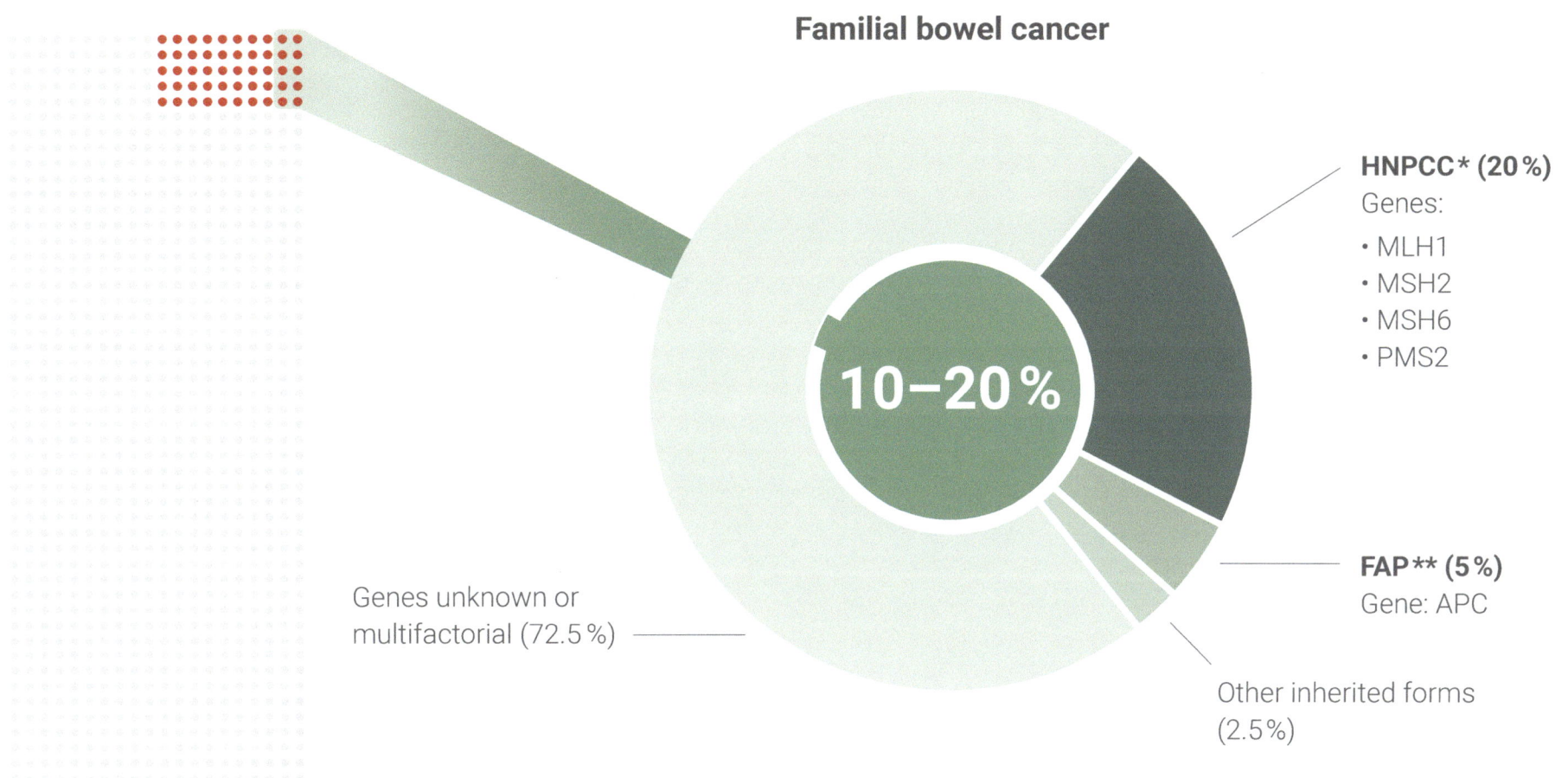

About 50 out of 1,000 people develop bowel cancer (1 out of 20, or 5 %)

Familial bowel cancer

10–20 %

HNPCC* (20 %)
Genes:
• MLH1
• MSH2
• MSH6
• PMS2

FAP** (5 %)
Gene: APC

Other inherited forms
(2.5 %)

Genes unknown or
multifactorial (72.5 %)

1,000 people

*HNPCC = hereditary nonpolyposis colorectal cancer
**FAP = familial adenomatous polyposis

HNPCC = hereditary nonpolyposis colorectal cancer

Revised Bethesda Criteria
At least **one** criterion must apply:

- Colorectal cancer diagnosed before age 50

- Synchronous/metachronous colorectal cancer or HNPCC-related cancers (endometrium, renal pelvis/ureter, small intestine, stomach, pancreas, bile duct, ovary, hepatobiliary system and brain – usually glioblastoma, sebaceous adenoma and kerato-acanthoma) regardless of age

- Colorectal cancer with the MSI-H (microsatellite instability-high) histology diagnosed before the age of 60

- Patient with colorectal cancer and at least one first-degree relative diagnosed with an HNPCC-related cancer before the age of 50

- Patient with colorectal cancer and at least two first- or second-degree relatives with HNPCC-related cancers (see above), regardless of age

Amsterdam II Criteria
All criteria must apply:

- Three or more family members with HNPCC-related cancer (colorectal, endometrial, small bowel, renal pelvis/ureter)

- One affected person is a first-degree relative of the other two affected individuals

- Disease in two or more successive generations

- At least one affected individual was diagnosed with cancer before the age of 50

- **F**amilial **a**denomatous **p**olyposis (FAP) has been excluded

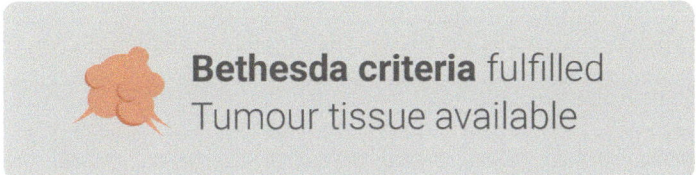

Bethesda criteria fulfilled
Tumour tissue available

Tumour tissue immunohistochemistry

| MLH1 **absent** | MSH2, MSH6, PMS2 **absent** | MLH1, MSH2, MSH6, PMS2 **present** |

BRAF mutation testing

HNPCC genetic testing

MSI (microsatellite instability) **testing**

| Mutated | Not mutated | | Unstable | Stable |

No genetic testing for HNPCC

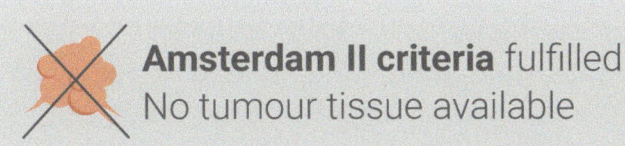

Amsterdam II criteria fulfilled
No tumour tissue available

No genetic testing for HNPCC

HNPCC: cancer spectrum and lifetime risks
Statistics for all HNPCC genes (German HNPCC Consortium data)

Cancer type	Risk
Colorectal cancer	30–60 % (women), 35–75 % (men)
Endometrial cancer	40–50 % (women)
Ovarian cancer	7–8 % (women)
Stomach cancer	1–6 %
Cancer of the renal pelvis / ureter	2–8 %
Bile duct cancer	1–4 %
Small bowel cancer	1–4 %
CNS cancers	2 %
Pancreatic cancer	4 %
Sebaceous gland tumours (Muir-Torre syndrome)	Depending on the affected gene

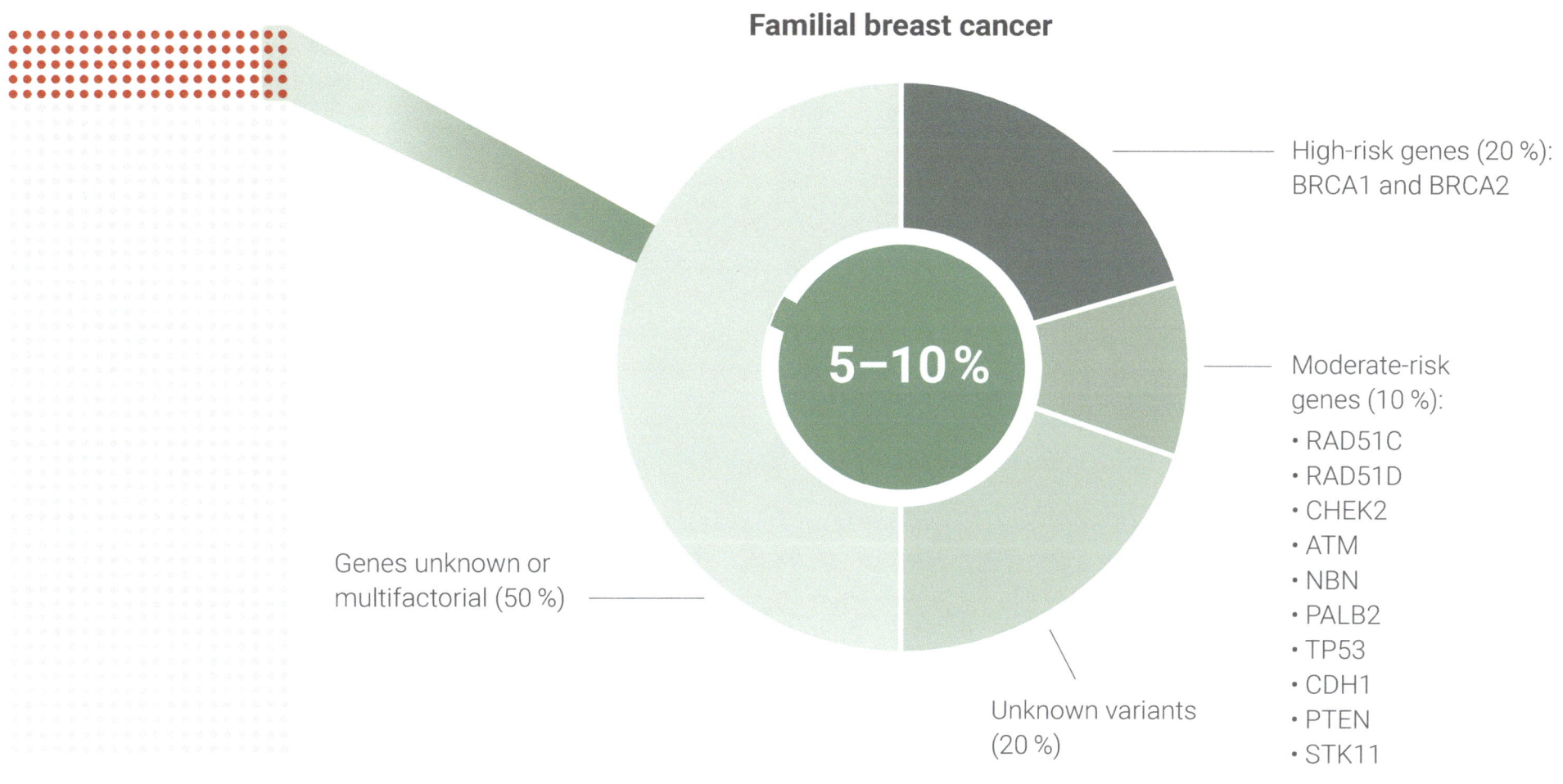

100 out of 1,000 women get breast cancer

Familial breast cancer

5–10 %

High-risk genes (20 %): BRCA1 and BRCA2

Moderate-risk genes (10 %):
• RAD51C
• RAD51D
• CHEK2
• ATM
• NBN
• PALB2
• TP53
• CDH1
• PTEN
• STK11

Unknown variants (20 %)

Genes unknown or multifactorial (50 %)

1,000 women

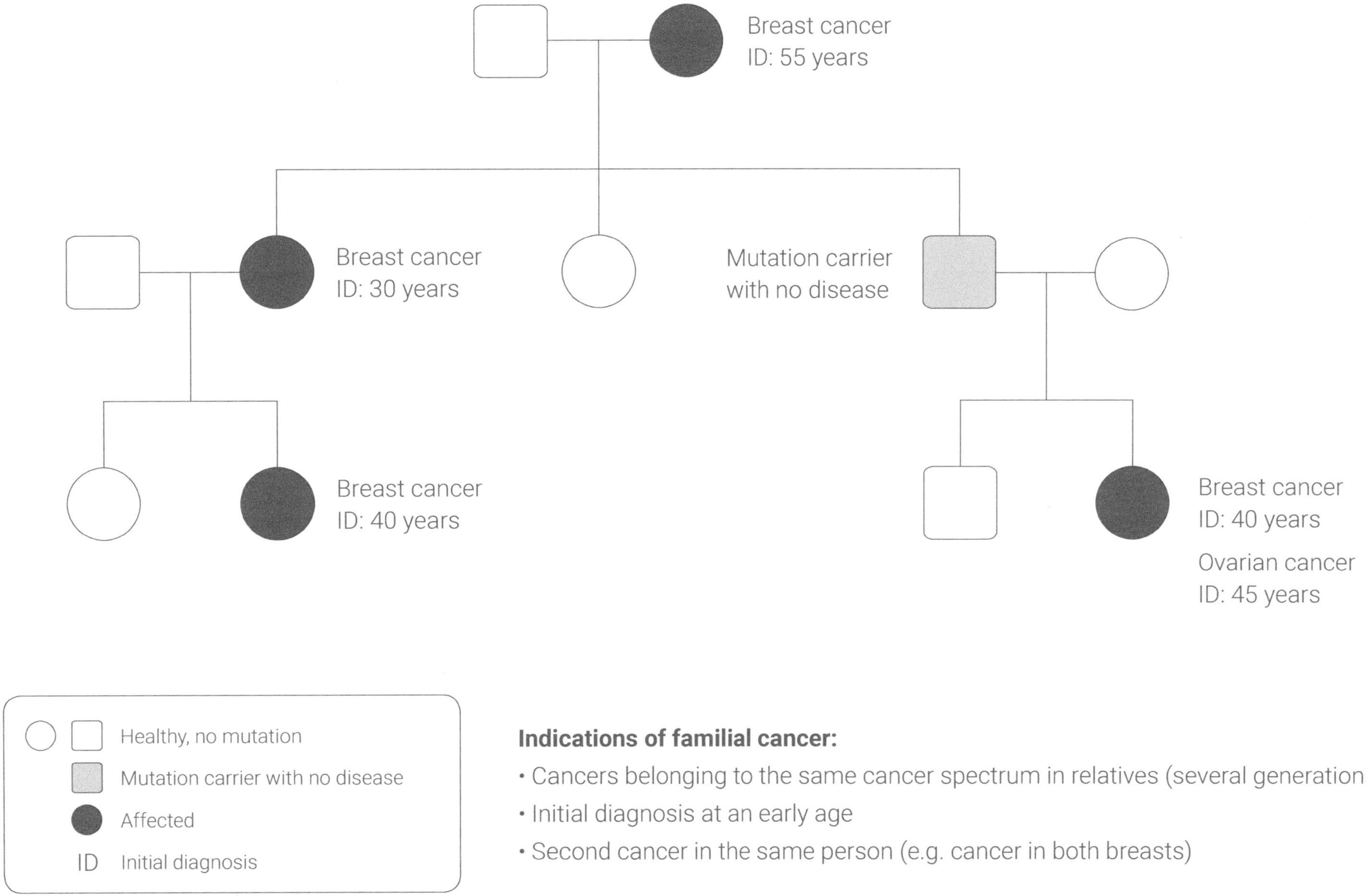

Breast cancer
ID: 55 years

Breast cancer
ID: 30 years

Mutation carrier
with no disease

Breast cancer
ID: 40 years

Breast cancer
ID: 40 years

Ovarian cancer
ID: 45 years

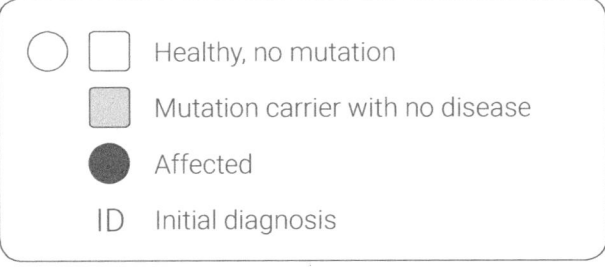

Healthy, no mutation

Mutation carrier with no disease

Affected

ID   Initial diagnosis

Indications of familial cancer:

· Cancers belonging to the same cancer spectrum in relatives (several generations)

· Initial diagnosis at an early age

· Second cancer in the same person (e.g. cancer in both breasts)

High-risk gene diagnostics advised when at least one of the following criteria applies:

- Three women of any age with breast cancer

- Two women with breast cancer, one of whom was diagnosed before the age of 51

- One woman with breast cancer diagnosed before the age of 36

- One woman with cancer in both breasts, the first diagnosed before the age of 51

- One woman with breast and ovarian cancer

- Two women with ovarian cancer

- One man with breast cancer and one woman with breast or ovarian cancer

Cancer spectrum	BRCA1	BRCA2	Risk in general population
Breast cancer	60–90 %	50–80 %	10 %
Ovarian cancer	20–40 %	10–30 %	1.5 %
Breast cancer (man)	1–2 %	5–10 %	0.1 %

Other types of cancer

Pancreatic cancer	1–3 %	2–7 %	0.5 %
Prostate	20–30 %	20–40 %	15 %
Malignant melanoma	1–2 %	1–2 %	1 %

G Common Disorders

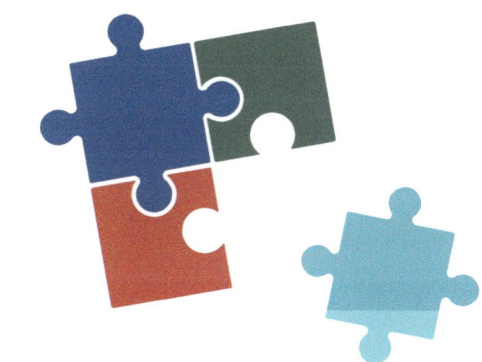

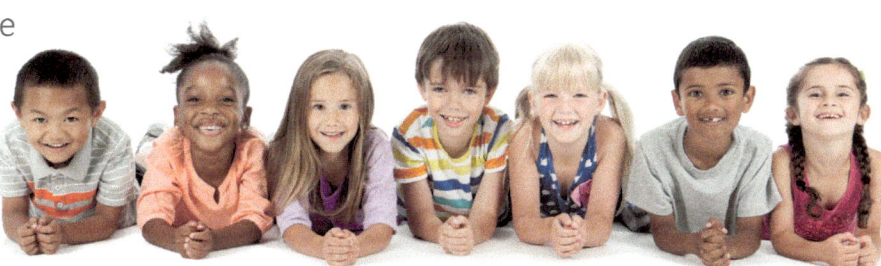

Child with developmental disorder or intellectual impairment

Clinical assessment

1. History:
- Pregnancy
- Development history
- Previous findings/cMRI

2. Pedigree:
- Other people affected?
- Inheritance pattern

3. Physical examination:
- Face ("one-look diagnosis")
- Skin, hair, hands, feet, etc.
- Examples (see G 37.2)

Clinical syndrome classification possible?

YES

Specific diagnostic workup:
- Chromosomes
- Gene(s)

NO

Basic diagnostics:
- Chromosomes
- Array CGH
- FMR1 gene (fragile X syndrome)

Further tests:
- Gene panel/exome

Genetic diagnosis
Enables conclusions regarding prognosis, treatment, prevention, inheritance, prenatal diagnostics

Malformations and dysmorphic features (examples)

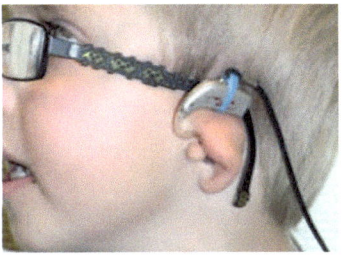
Ear malformation

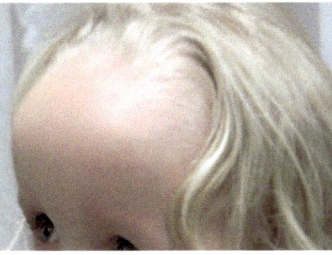
High forehead

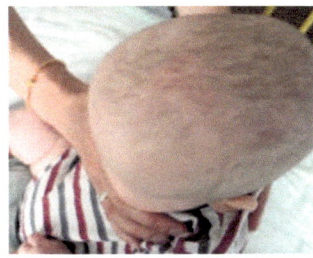
Scaphocephaly (long, narrow head)

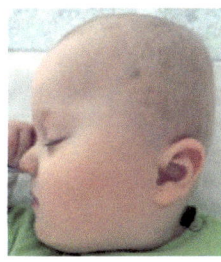
Brachycephaly

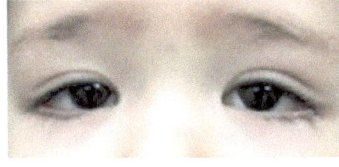
Eyes that slant downwards

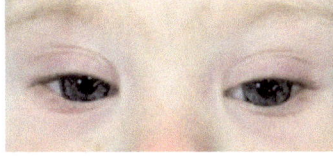
Eyes that slant upwards
Epicanthus (fold of skin over inner angle of the eye)

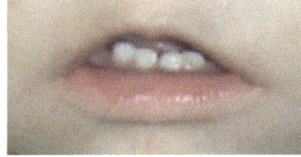
Thin upper lip
Drooping corners of the mouth

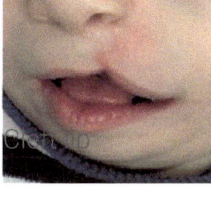

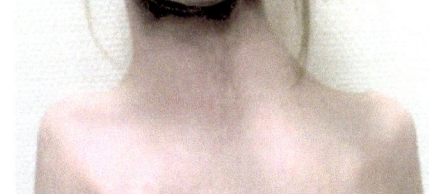
Pterygium colli (webbed neck)

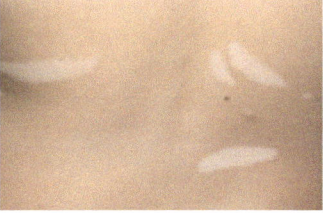
Café-au-lait spot
Neurofibroma

White spots

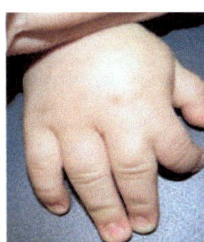
Single transverse palmar crease

Syndactyly

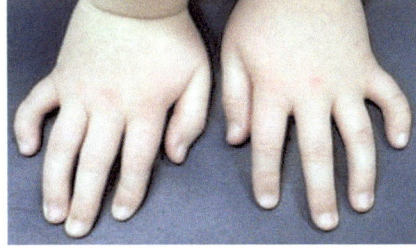
Clinodactyly

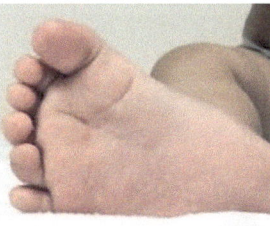
Hexadactyly

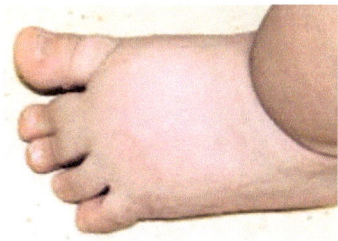
Syndactyly

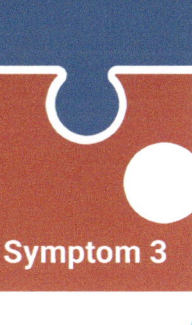

Symptom 1 Symptom 2

Symptom 3

?

Syndrome diagnosis

Genetic diagnostics

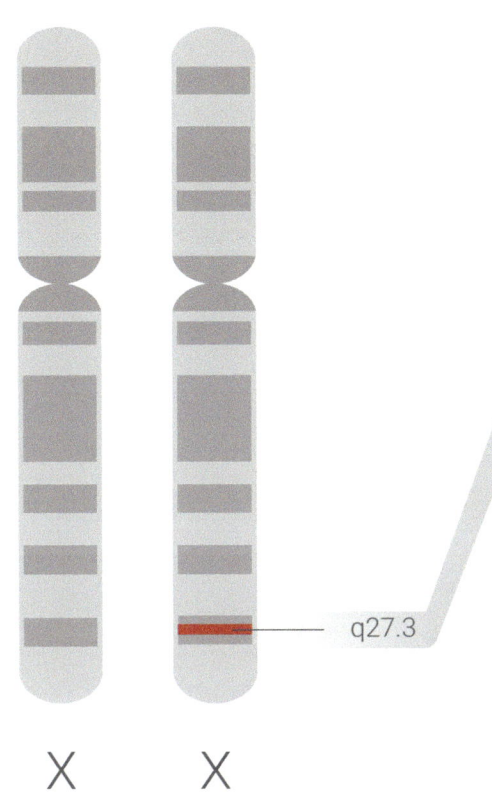

CGG repeat in FMR1 gene (fragile X mental retardation 1):

...CGG-CGG-CGG-CGG-CGG-CGG-CGG-CGG-CGG-CGG...

Normal: CGG < 45

Grey area: CGG 45-54

Premutation: CGG 55-200

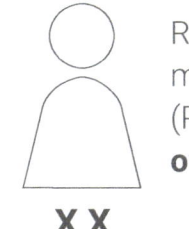

Risk of early menopause (POF = **p**remature **o**varian **f**ailure)

X X

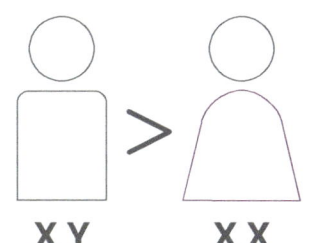

>

Risk of late-onset FXTAS (fragile X-associated tremor/ataxia syndrome)

X Y   X X

Full mutation: CGG > 200 ➡ **Fragile X syndrome**

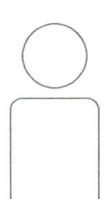

100 % intellectual disability

X Y

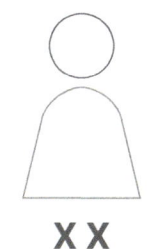

40 % normal development
30 % learning difficulties
30 % intellectual disability

X X

q27.3

X   X

Fragile X syndrome

Common cause of intellectual disability in boys (1:4,000) and girls (1:6,000)

Mother with premutation

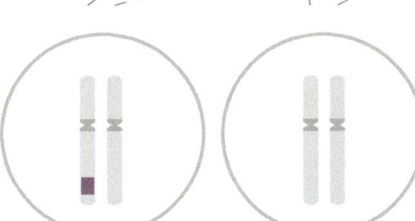

X X   X Y

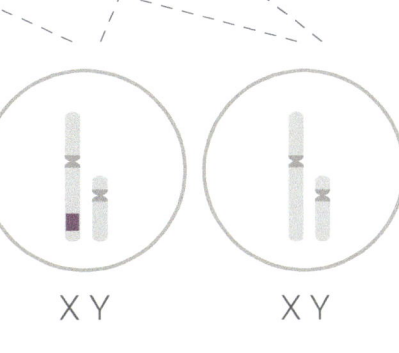

X X   X X   X Y   X Y

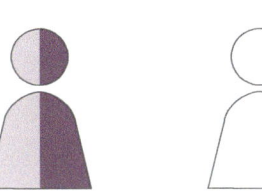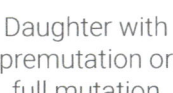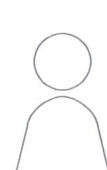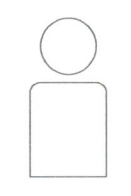

Daughter with premutation or full mutation

Healthy daughter

Son with premutation or full mutation

Healthy son

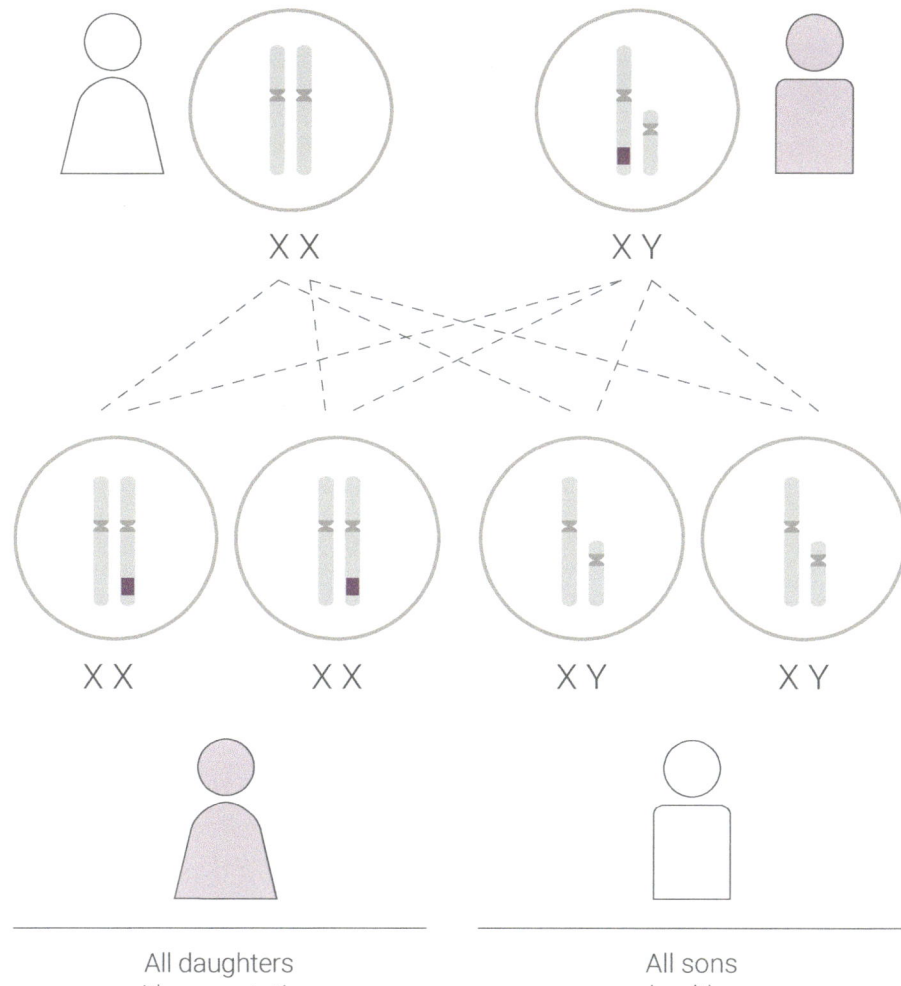

Father with premutation

X X   X Y

X X   X X   X Y   X Y

All daughters with premutation

All sons healthy

Pedigree example:

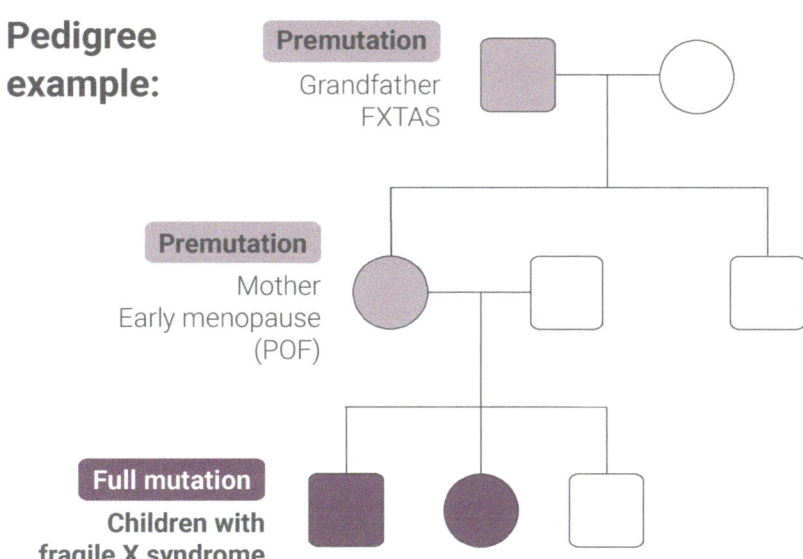

Premutation
Grandfather
FXTAS

Premutation
Mother
Early menopause
(POF)

Full mutation

**Children with
fragile X syndrome**

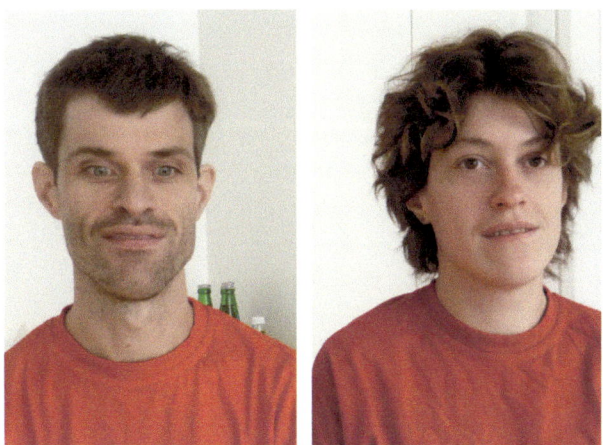

Brother and sister with fragile X syndrome

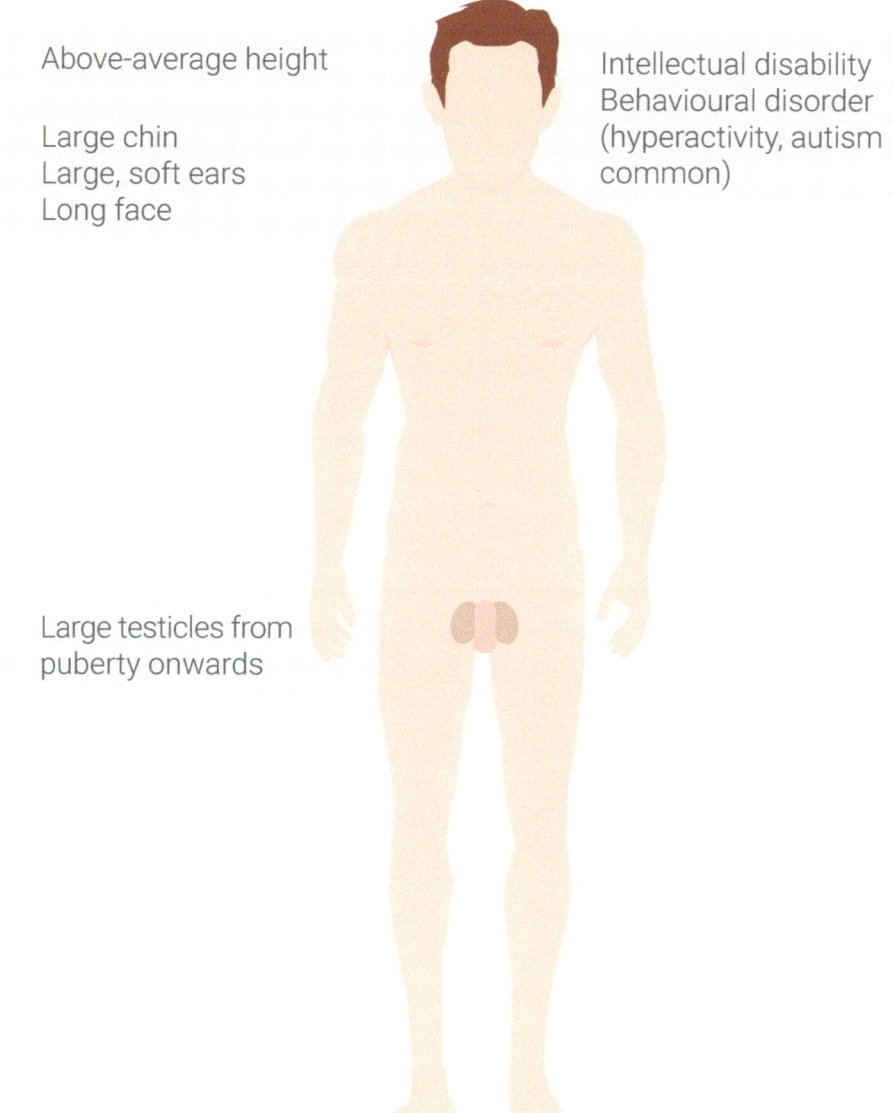

Above-average height

Large chin
Large, soft ears
Long face

Intellectual disability
Behavioural disorder
(hyperactivity, autism
common)

Large testicles from
puberty onwards

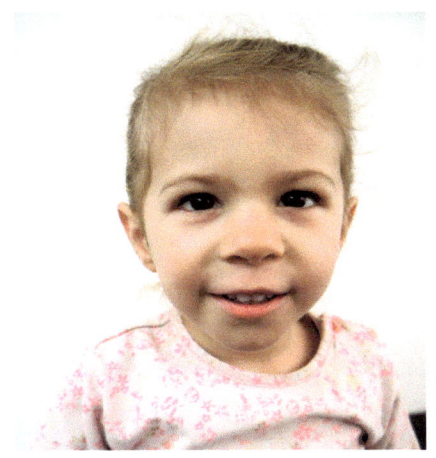

Girl (age 3)
with Prader-Willi syndrome

Incidence:

1:10,000 girls and boys

Therapy:

• Dietary control (lock food away if necessary)

• Promote psychomotor skills

• Growth hormone

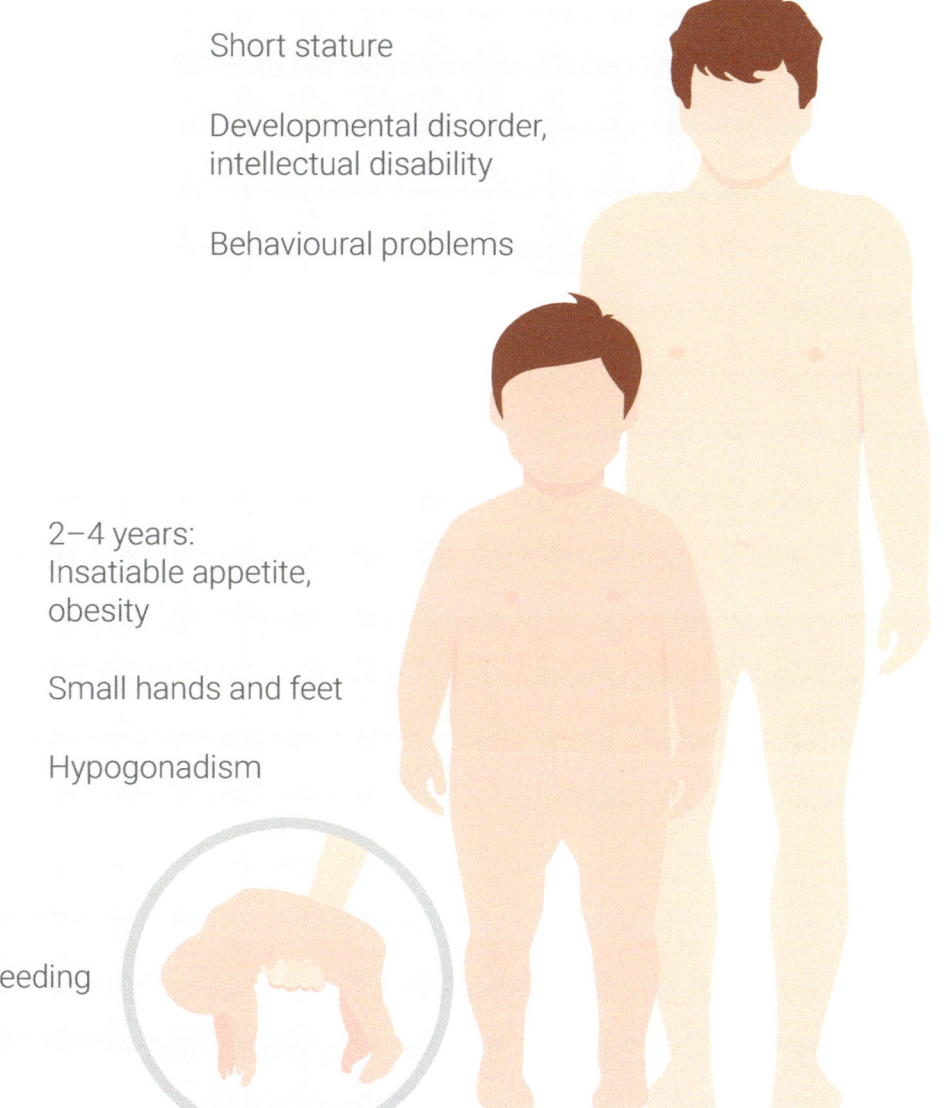

Short stature

Developmental disorder,
intellectual disability

Behavioural problems

2–4 years:
Insatiable appetite,
obesity

Small hands and feet

Hypogonadism

Weak muscle tone

Poor feeding: tube feeding
is often necessary

Normal:
Paternally imprinted genes are active

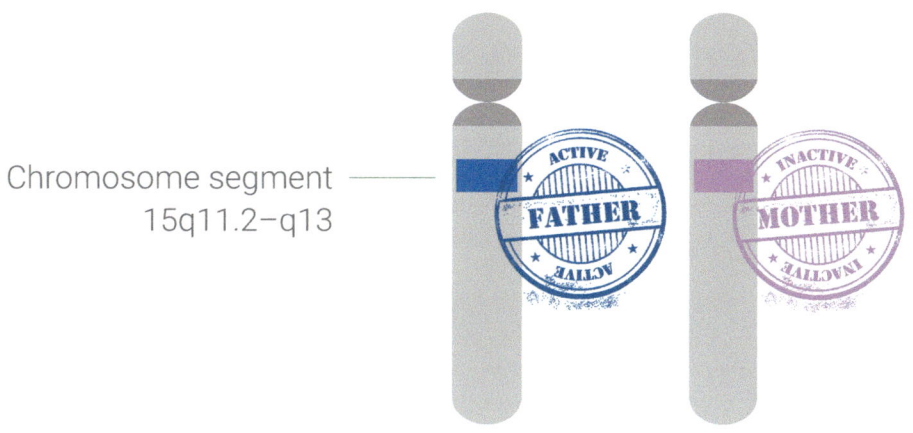

Chromosome segment
15q11.2–q13

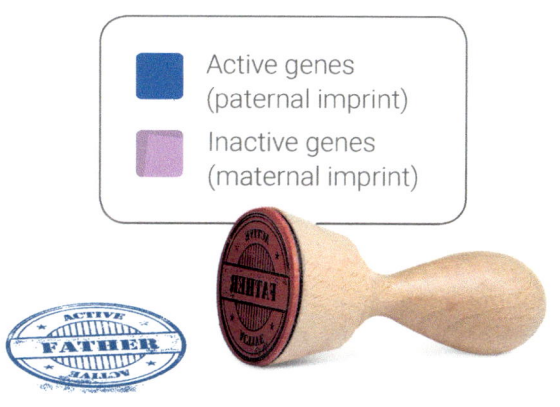

Active genes
(paternal imprint)

Inactive genes
(maternal imprint)

Prader-Willi syndrome:
Loss of function of paternally imprinted genes

Deletion

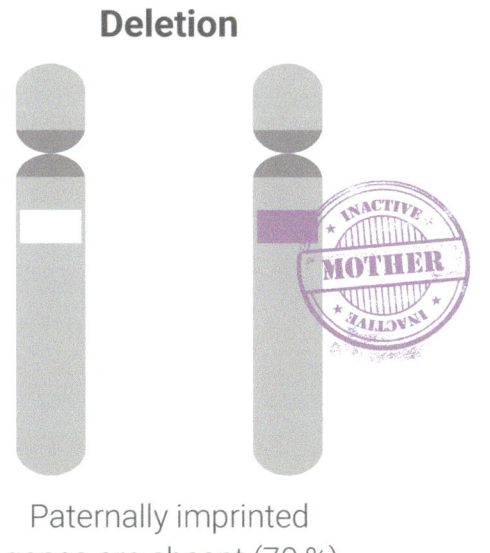

Paternally imprinted
genes are absent (70 %)

Maternal UPD 15

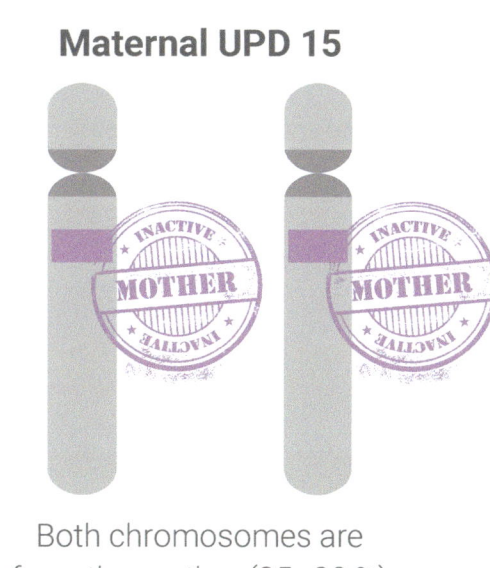

Both chromosomes are
from the mother (25–30 %)

Imprinting defect

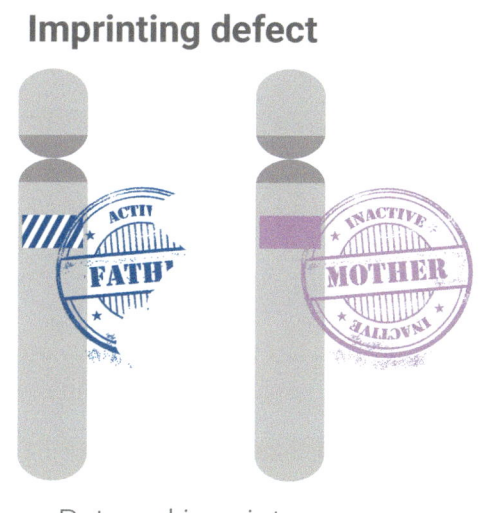

Paternal imprint
is non-functioning (< 1 %)

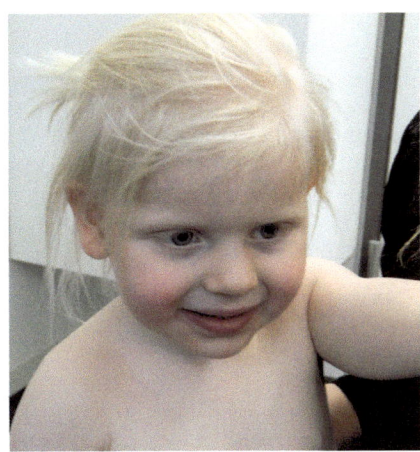

Girl (age 2)
with Angelman syndrome

Incidence:

1:15,000–20,000 girls and boys

Therapy:

• Symptomatic (epilepsy in particular)

• Promote psychomotor skills

Small head

Severe language
development disorder

Drooling

Light-coloured hair
and pale skin, blue eyes
are common

Happy personality

Hyperactivity

Ataxia

Intellectual disability

Epilepsy (specific
EEG abnormality)

Squint

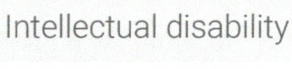

Normal:

Maternally imprinted genes are active

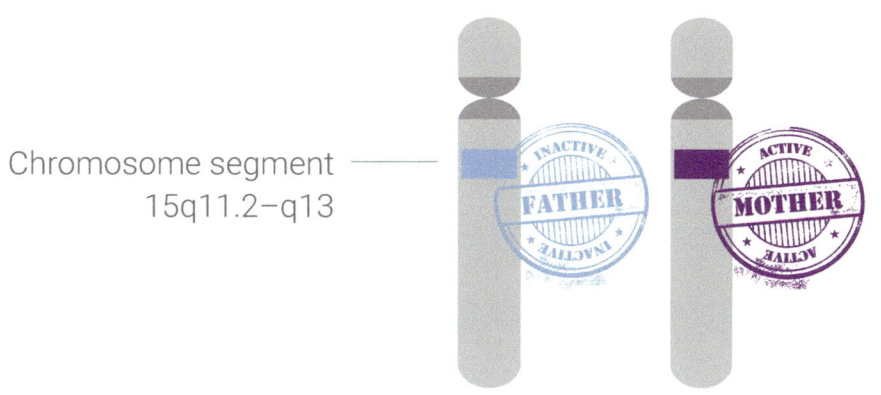

Chromosome segment
15q11.2–q13

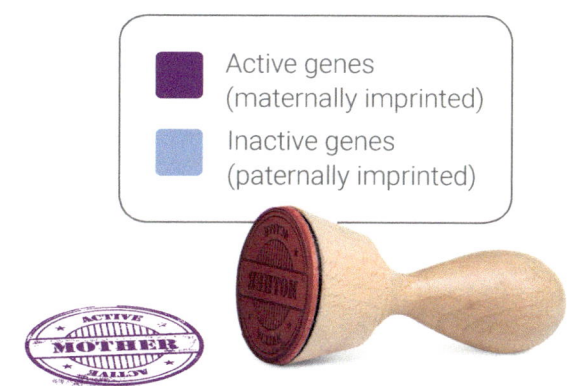

- ■ Active genes
  (maternally imprinted)
- ■ Inactive genes
  (paternally imprinted)

Angelman syndrome:

Loss of function of maternally imprinted genes

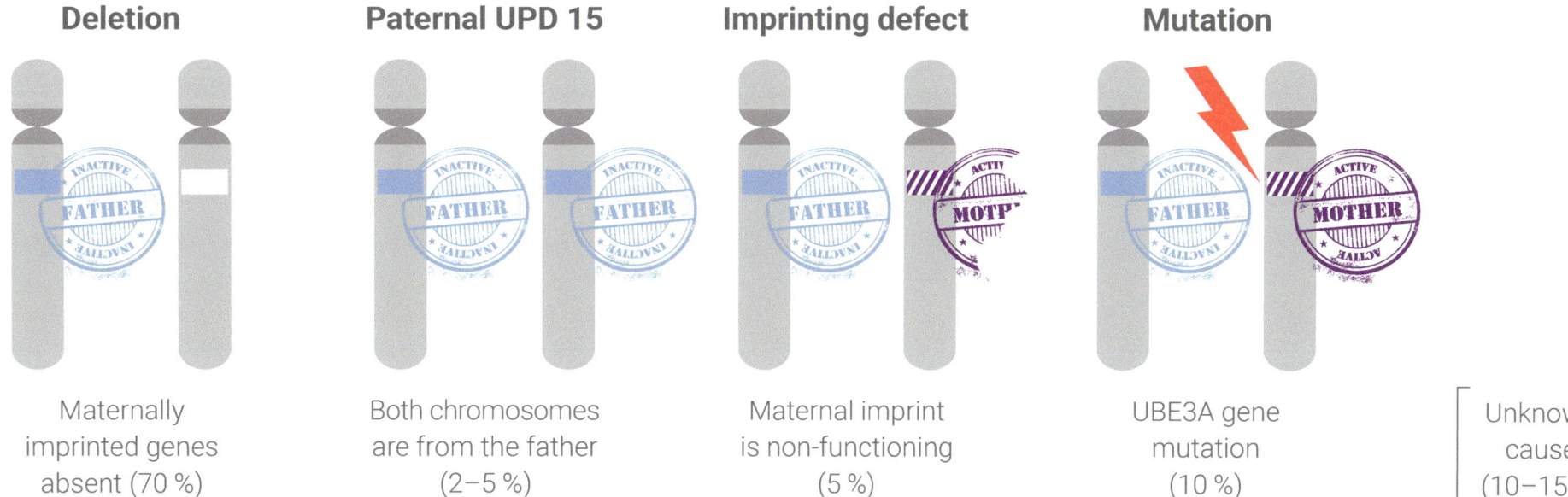

Deletion

Maternally
imprinted genes
absent (70 %)

Paternal UPD 15

Both chromosomes
are from the father
(2–5 %)

Imprinting defect

Maternal imprint
is non-functioning
(5 %)

Mutation

UBE3A gene
mutation
(10 %)

Unknown
cause
(10–15 %)

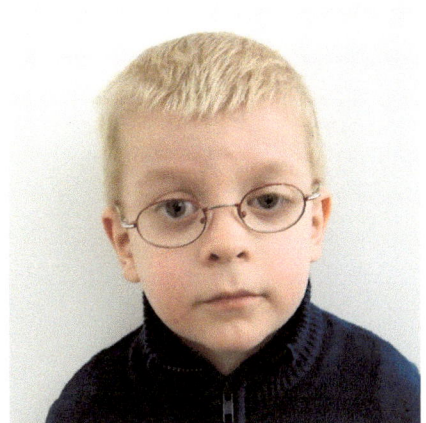

Boy (age 5) with
Noonan syndrome

Incidence:

Approx. 1:2,000 boys and girls

Inheritance:

Autosomal dominant

Genes:

50 %: PTPN11

30 %: RAF1, SOS1, KRAS, RIT1,
SHOC2, BRAF, CBL,
HRAS, MAP2K1/MEK1,
MAP2K2/MEK2

20 %: Hitherto unknown genes

Mild developmental delay (common)
Learning difficulties in about 30–50 %

Face:
• Large head
• High, broad forehead
• Wide-set eyes
• Epicanthus (fold of skin
over the inner angle of the eye)
• Eyes that slant downwards
with drooping eyelids (ptosis)
• Webbed neck (pterygium colli)
• Low-set ears

Renal anomalies

Undescended testicles (boys)

Therapy:

• Growth hormone may help

• Promote psychomotor skills

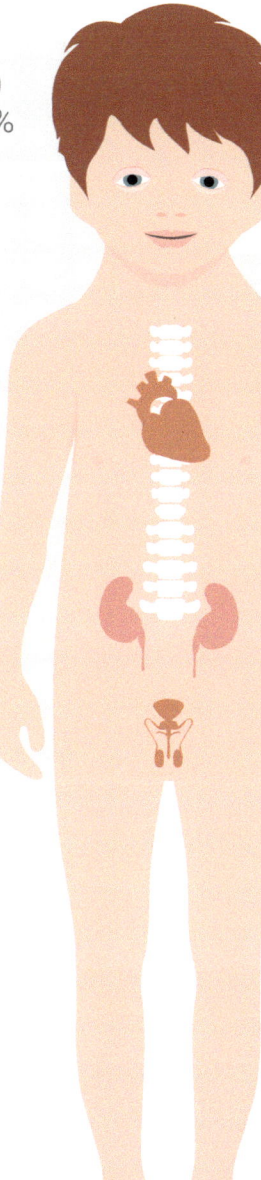

Short stature

Heart:
• Pulmonary stenosis
is common
• Atrial septal defect
• Hypertrophic
cardiomyopathy

Sunken or protruding
chest, nipples far apart

Scoliosis

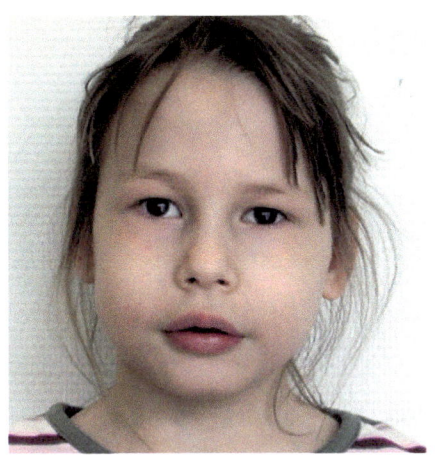

Girl (age 8) with
microdeletion syndrome 22q11

Incidence:

Approx. 1:4,000 girls and boys

Synonyms:

Microdeletion syndrome 22q11

DiGeorge syndrome

Velocardiofacial syndrome (VCFS)

Shprintzen syndrome (formerly CATCH 22)

Brain:
- Developmental disorder
- Learning difficulties
- Increased risk of psychosis in adulthood (approx. 10–20 %)

Cleft palate (nasal speech)

Weak immune system
Thymus hypoplasia or aplasia

Malformation of other organs, e.g. kidneys

Expression is highly variable

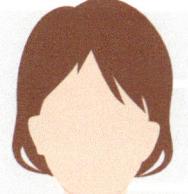
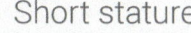
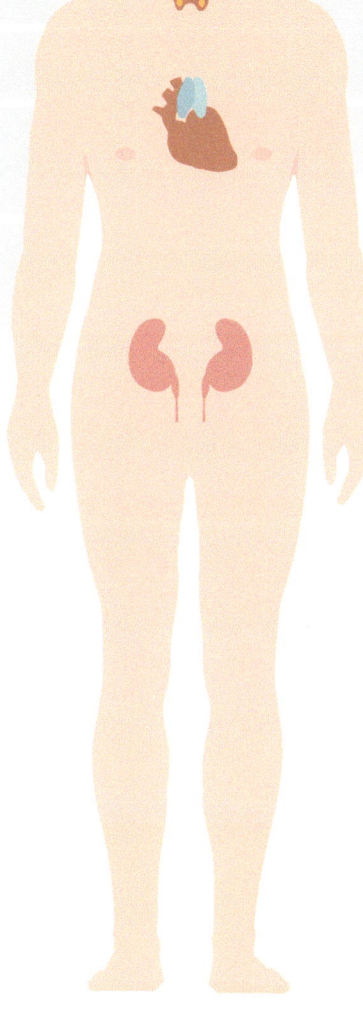

Short stature

Prominent ears
Long face

Parathyroid abnormalities (low calcium)

Heart defects

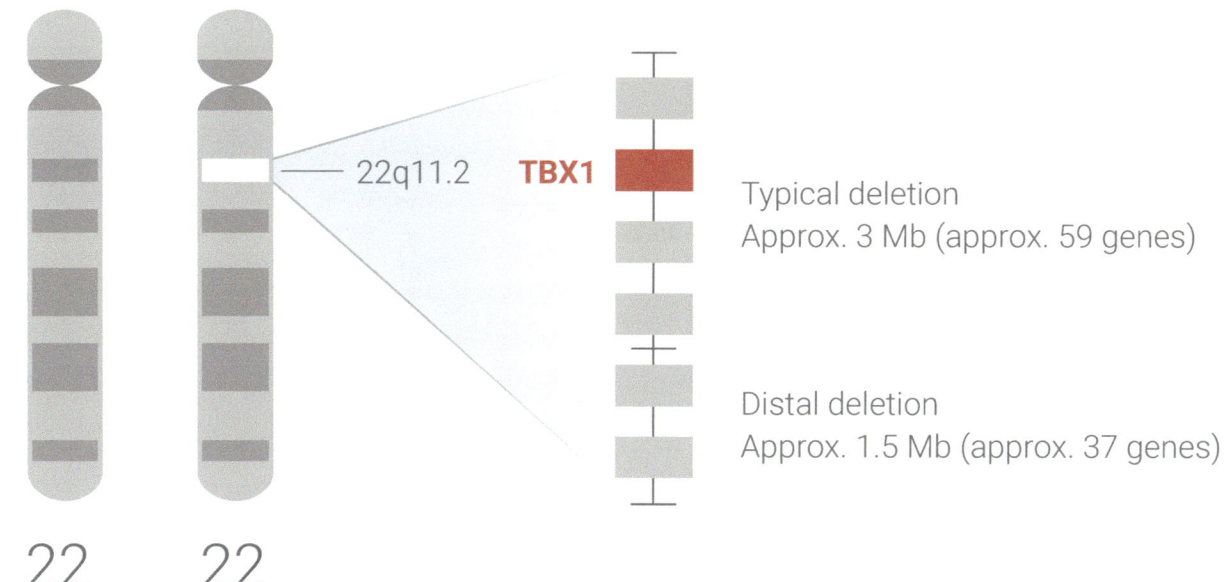

22q11.2

TBX1

Typical deletion
Approx. 3 Mb (approx. 59 genes)

Distal deletion
Approx. 1.5 Mb (approx. 37 genes)

22   22

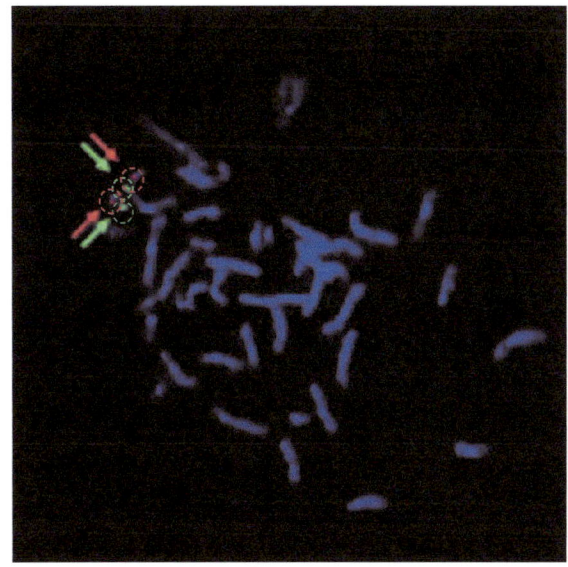

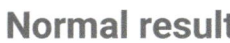

Normal result

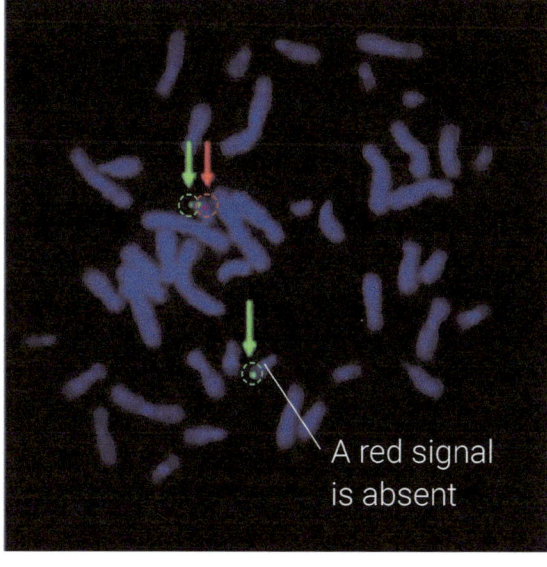

A red signal
is absent

Microdeletion 22q11

↓ Target probe 22q11

↓ Control probe

FISH
(**f**luorescent **i**n **s**itu **h**ybridisation)

Array CGH (microdeletion 22q11)

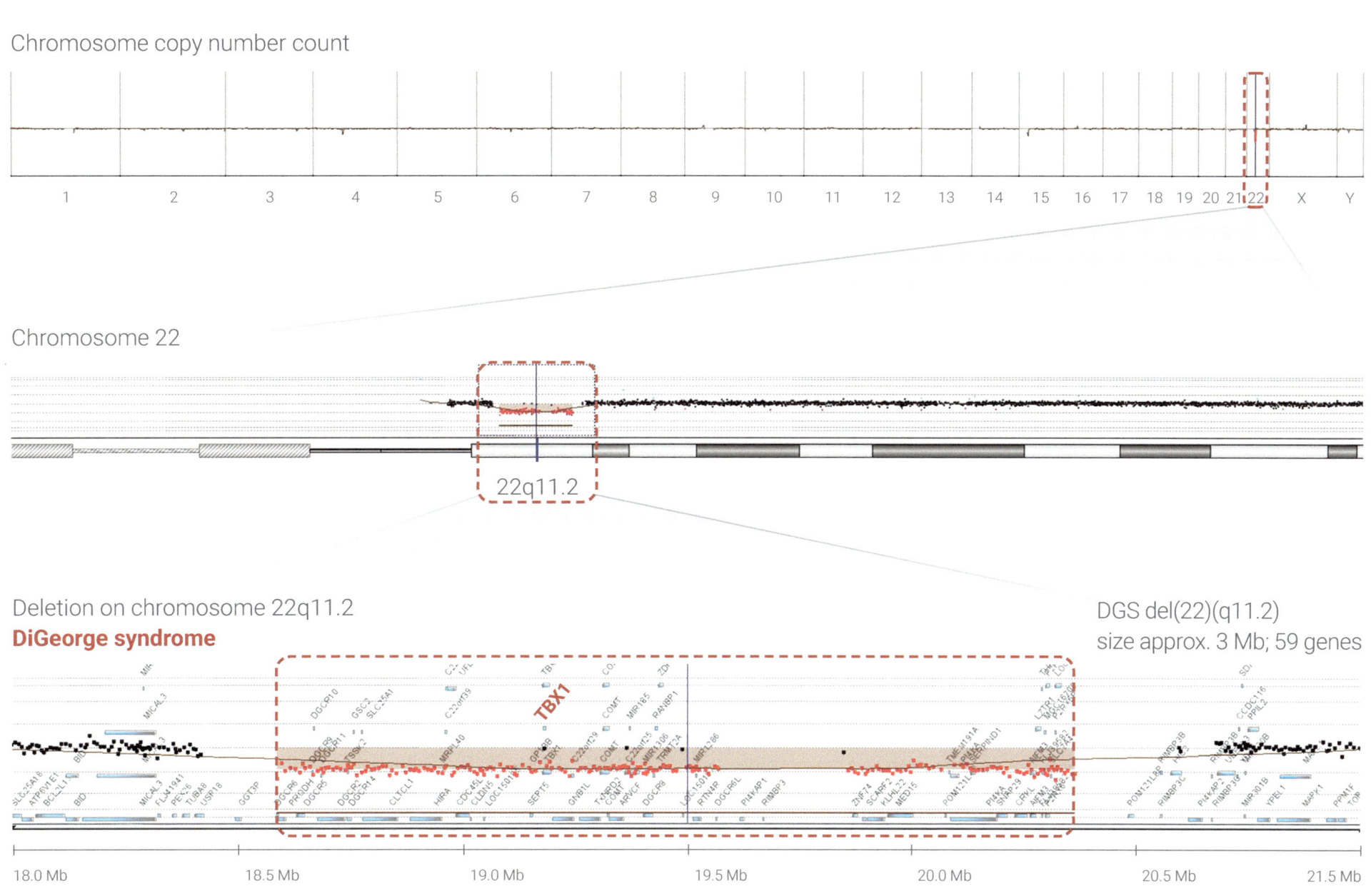

Chromosome copy number count

Chromosome 22

22q11.2

Deletion on chromosome 22q11.2
DiGeorge syndrome

TBX1

DGS del(22)(q11.2)
size approx. 3 Mb; 59 genes

18.0 Mb   18.5 Mb   19.0 Mb   19.5 Mb   20.0 Mb   20.5 Mb   21.5 Mb

Neurofibromatosis type 1: von Recklinghausen disease

Diagnostic criteria

(based on NIH Consensus Statement, 1988)

- ≥ 6 café-au-lait spots > 0.5 cm
  (before puberty) or > 1.5 cm (after puberty)

- ≥ 2 neurofibromas or > 1 plexiform
  neurofibroma

- Freckling (inguinal or axillary)

- Optic nerve glioma

- Lisch nodules

- Bone symptoms, e.g. congenital
  pseudarthrosis of tibia

- At least one first-degree relative with
  neurofibromatosis type 1

Incidence: Approx. 1:3,000

Gene: NF1 (neurofibromin, chromosome 17)

Inheritance:
Autosomal dominant
50 % new mutations

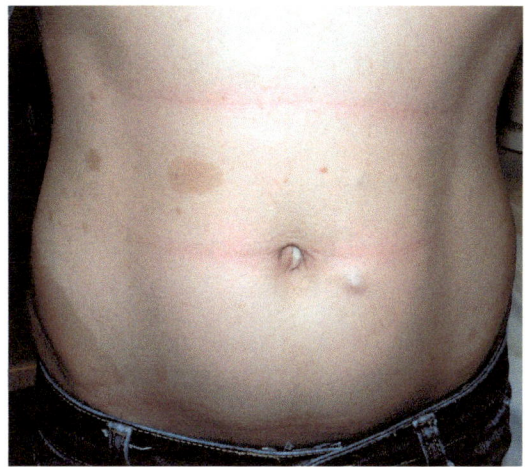

Neurofibroma and café-au-lait spots

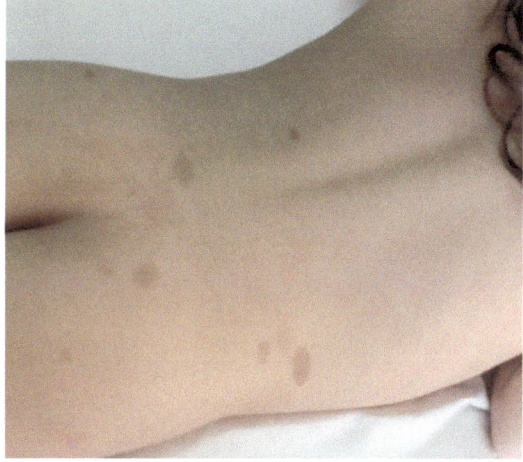

Café-au-lait spots

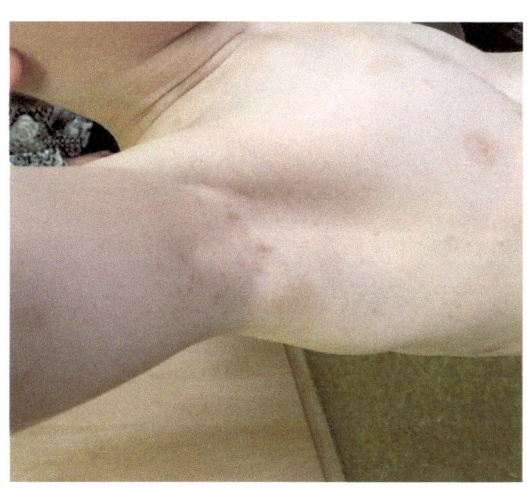

Freckling

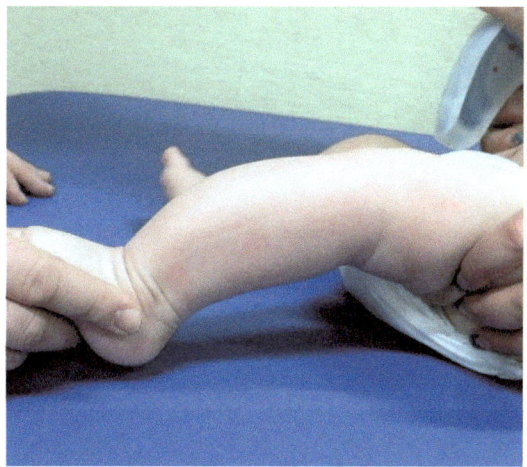

Pseudarthrosis of tibia

Neurofibromatosis type 2

Various clinical manifestations are possible:

1. Multiple bilateral schwannomas of the cranial nerves, especially the eighth cranial nerve (clinical features: hearing disorder, tinnitus, facial nerve paralysis) 50 % have additional CNS tumours, especially meningeoma

2. Subcutaneous schwannomas and neurofibromas

3. Eyes: cataract (clouding of the lens) from childhood

Possible additional symptoms:

• Café-au-lait spots

• Increased risk of neoplasms, in particular astrocytoma, oligodendroglioma and ependymomas

Incidence: Approx. 1:50,000

Gene: NF2 (schwannomin, chromosome 22)

Inheritance:

Autosomal dominant

50 % new mutations

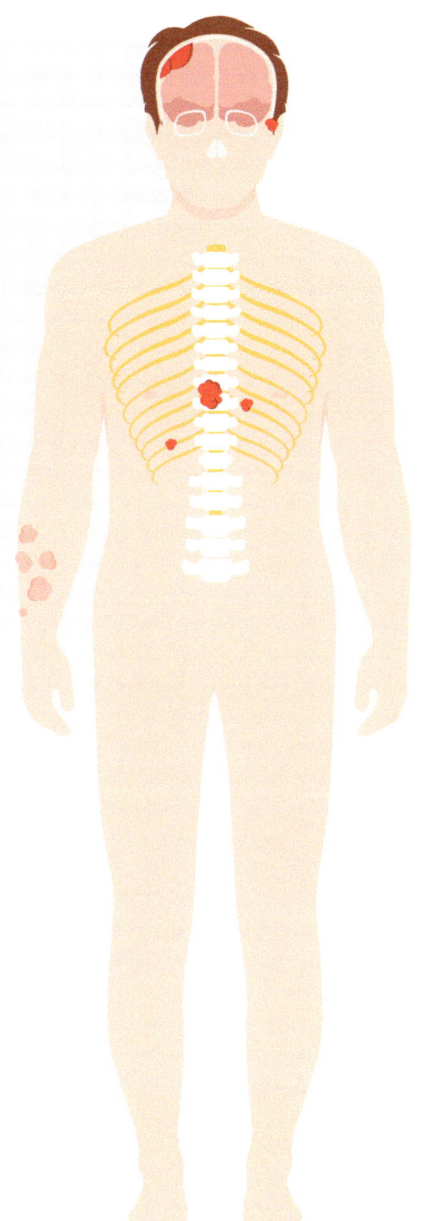

Meningeoma

Early-onset cataracts

Cranial nerve schwannoma (commonly involving the hearing nerve)
Hearing loss/deafness

Spinal cord and peripheral nerve tumours

Skin tumours (mainly benign)

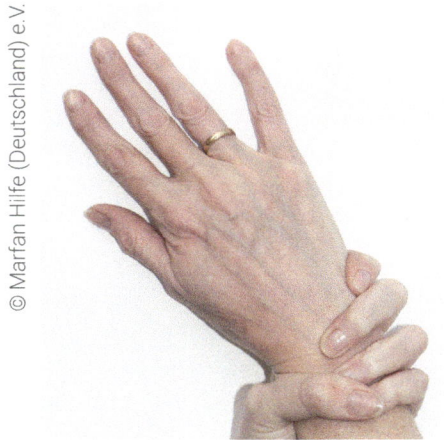

Positive wrist sign in a woman with Marfan syndrome

Incidence:

Approx. 1:5,000–10,000

Inheritance:

Autosomal dominant

Approx. 30 % new mutations

Connective tissue defect due to mutation in the FBN1 gene (fibrillin, chromosome 15)

Rare: TGFBR1 or TGFBR2 gene

Therapy:

Beta-blockers may help (prevention)

Eye:
severe short-sightedness (myopia), lens dislocation, increased risk of retinal detachment, glaucoma and early-onset cataracts

Skeletal:
sunken or protruding chest, scoliosis

Heart:
aortic aneurysm and aortic dissection (tear), valve changes

Lumbosacral dural ectasia

Protrusio acetabuli (x-ray)

Long fingers (arachnodactyly)

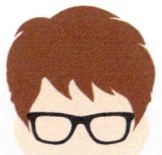

Above-average height

High-arched palate and narrow jaw (crowding of teeth)

Lungs: risk of pneumothorax

Long limbs

Flat feet, pes planovalgus

© Marfan Hilfe (Deutschland) e.V.

Clinical score (based on the revised Ghent nosology)

Characteristic	Points
Wrist AND thumb sign positive	3
Wrist OR thumb sign positive	1
Protruding chest (pectus carinatum)	2
Pectus excavatum or thoracic asymmetry	1
Pes valgus	2
Pes planus	1
Pneumothorax (ruptured lung)	2
Dural ectasia	2
Protrusio acetabuli (deformity of the acetabulum of the hip joint)	2
Upper to lower segment ratio reduced and arm span/body height ratio > 1.05	1
Scoliosis or thoracolumbar kyphosis	1
Reduced elbow extension (< 170°)	1
Facial features (at least 3 of 5): • Long, narrow skull • Downward slanted eyes • Deep-set eyes • Small and recessed lower jaw • Underdeveloped cheekbones	1
Stretch marks on the skin	1
Short-sightedness (myopia) > 3 dioptres	1
Mitral valve prolapse	1
Total clinical score	

Clinical diagnosis of Marfan syndrome

Family history **negative** for Marfan syndrome

At least **one** criterion must apply:

• Aortic root dilatation (aneurysm) with Z score ≥ 2 and one additional criterion:

 + Ectopia lentis

 + Mutation in FBN1 gene

 + Clinical score ≥ 7

• Ectopia lentis and evidence of FBN1 mutation known to be associated with aortic root dilatation

Family history **positive** for Marfan syndrome

At least **one** criterion must apply:

• Ectopia lentis

• Clinical score ≥ 7

• Aortic root dilatation (Z score > 3 under 20 years of age; Z score > 2 over 20 years of age)

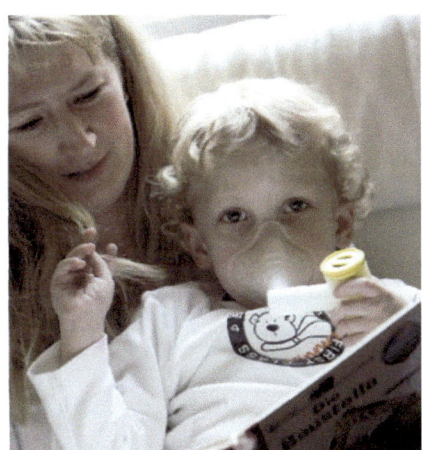

Boy (age 3) with cystic fibrosis
having inhalation therapy

Incidence:

1:2,500 (Central Europe).
One out of 25 people is a carrier.

Therapy:

• Inhalation.

• Physical therapy.

• Digestive enzymes (capsules).

• Antibiotics.

• Gene therapy (experimental).

• Heart + lung transplant surgery
  may be an option.

Failure to thrive/short stature

Sinusitis

Lungs:
chronic cough,
inflammation,
fibrosis (long term)

Liver/bile ducts:
bile duct obstruction,
cirrhosis of the liver

Vas deferens obstruction:
congenital bilateral aplasia
of the vas deferens (= CBAVD)
leads to infertility

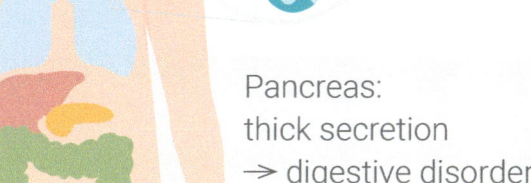

Pancreas:
thick secretion
→ digestive disorder

Bowel obstruction
in neonates
(= meconium ileus)

Mutation in the CFTR gene (cystic fibrosis transmembrane regulator)

Severe mutation: e.g. F508del
= most common mutation (approx. 70 %)

There is **loss** of amino acid F (phenylalanine).

Mild mutation: e.g. A455E

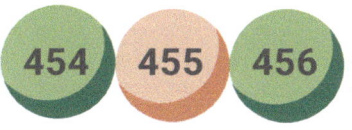

A (alanine) is **substituted** by E (glutamic acid).

Defective chloride channel (CFTR)

Healthy

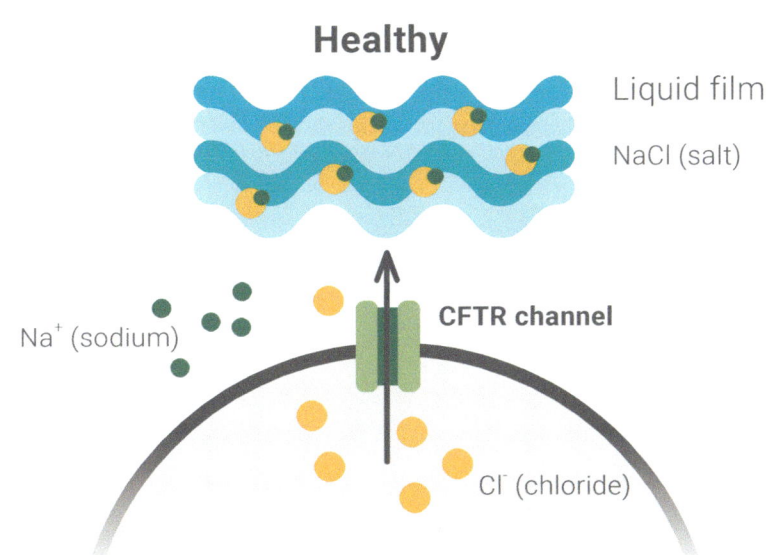

Liquid film

NaCl (salt)

Na$^+$ (sodium)

CFTR channel

Cl$^-$ (chloride)

Cystic fibrosis

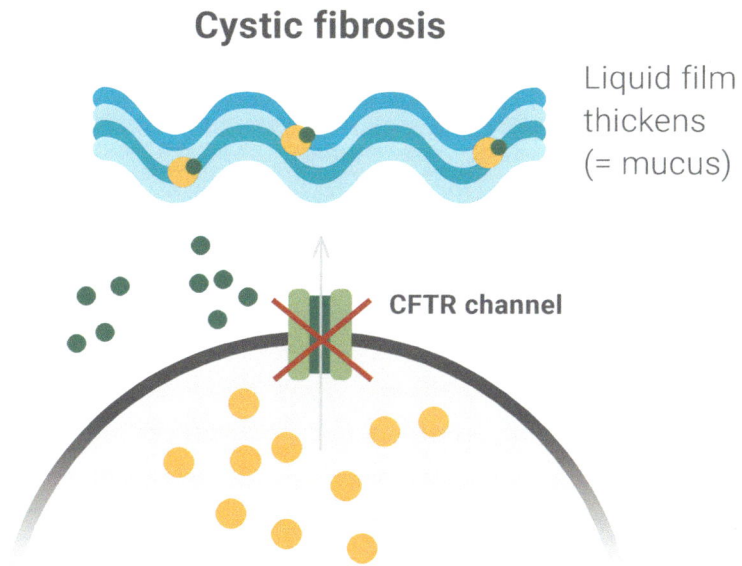

Liquid film thickens (= mucus)

CFTR channel

Autosomal recessive inheritance
One out of 25 people is a carrier.

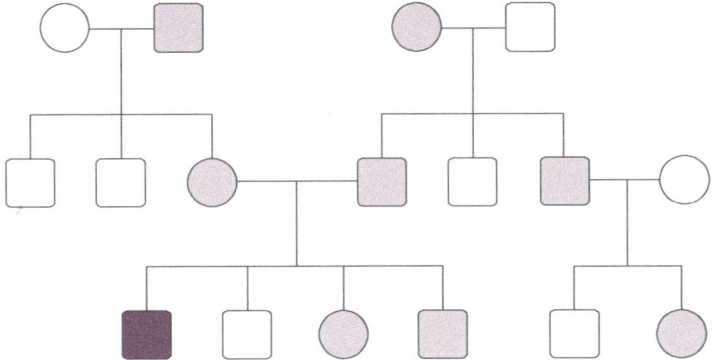

Father:
healthy carrier
for cystic fibrosis

Mother:
healthy carrier
for cystic fibrosis

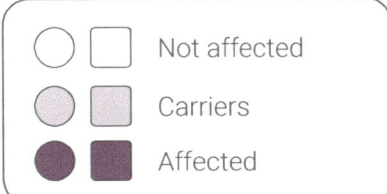

Not affected

Carriers

Affected

Gametes

Fertilisation

Characteristics

- Both parents are carriers: 25 % risk of an affected child.
- Girls and boys are equally affected.
- Affected individuals commonly occur in one generation only.
- There is an increased risk of affected offspring in consanguineous marriages.

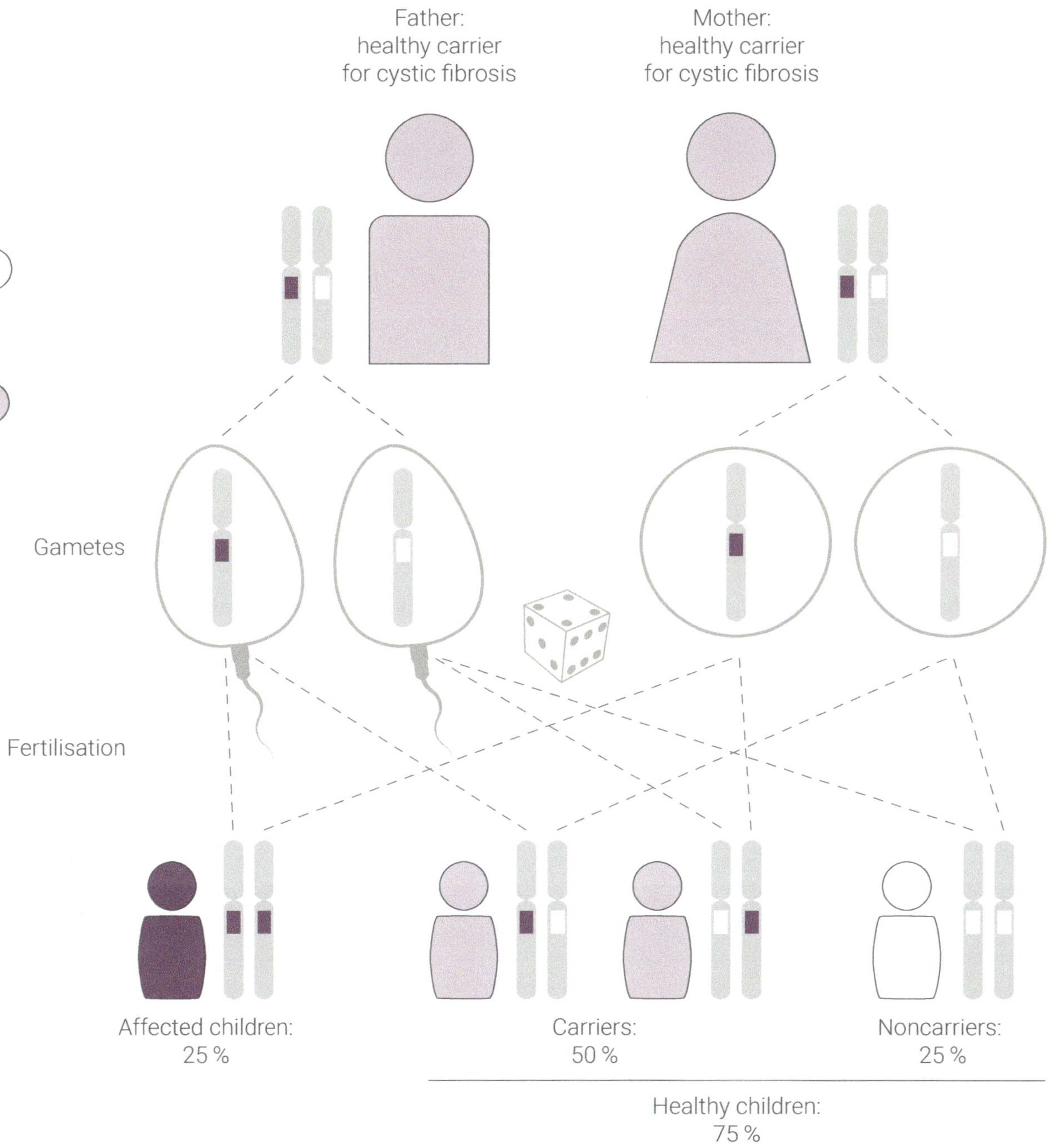

Affected children:
25 %

Carriers:
50 %

Noncarriers:
25 %

Healthy children:
75 %

Congenital metabolic disorders
(detected in neonatal metabolic screening)

Disorder	Frequency	Symptoms	Treatment
Phenylketonuria	1:10,000	Epilepsy, spasticity, intellectual disability	Special low-phenylalanine diet
Adrenogenital syndrome	1:10,000	Virilisation in girls, fatal outcome in boys and girls possible due to loss of salts and cortisol deficiency	Corticoids
MCAD deficiency	1:10,000	Metabolic crises with hypoglycaemia, liver failure, coma	Avoid periods of hunger, carnitine may help
Galactosaemia	1:40,000	Liver failure, physical and intellectual disability, cataract	Special galactose-free diet
Isovaleric acidaemia	1:50,000	Vomiting, coma, distinctive odour of sweaty feet, intellectual disability	Special diet, amino acids
Biotinidase deficiency	1:80,000	Skin changes, metabolic crises, intellectual disability	Biotin
LCHAD and VLCAD deficiency	1:80,000	Metabolic crises secondary to hypoglycaemia, coma, weak muscle tone and weak heart	Avoid periods of hunger, special diet
Glutaric aciduria type I	1:80,000	Metabolic crises, impaired mobility, large head	Special diet, carnitine
Carnitine metabolism disorders	1:100,000	Metabolic crises with hypoglycaemia, coma, weak heart	Avoid periods of hunger, special diet
Maple syrup disease	1:200,000	Coma, fatal outcome or intellectual disability	Special diet

Autosomal recessive inheritance

(underlies most metabolic disorders)

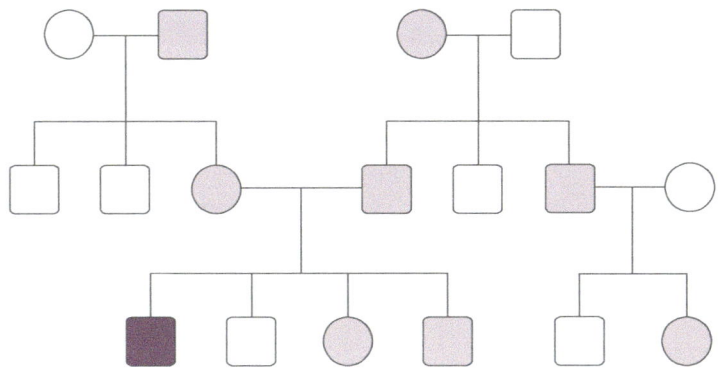

Father:
healthy carrier

Mother:
healthy carrier

Gametes

Fertilisation

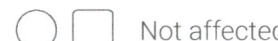	Not affected
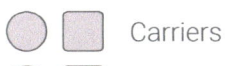	Carriers
	Affected

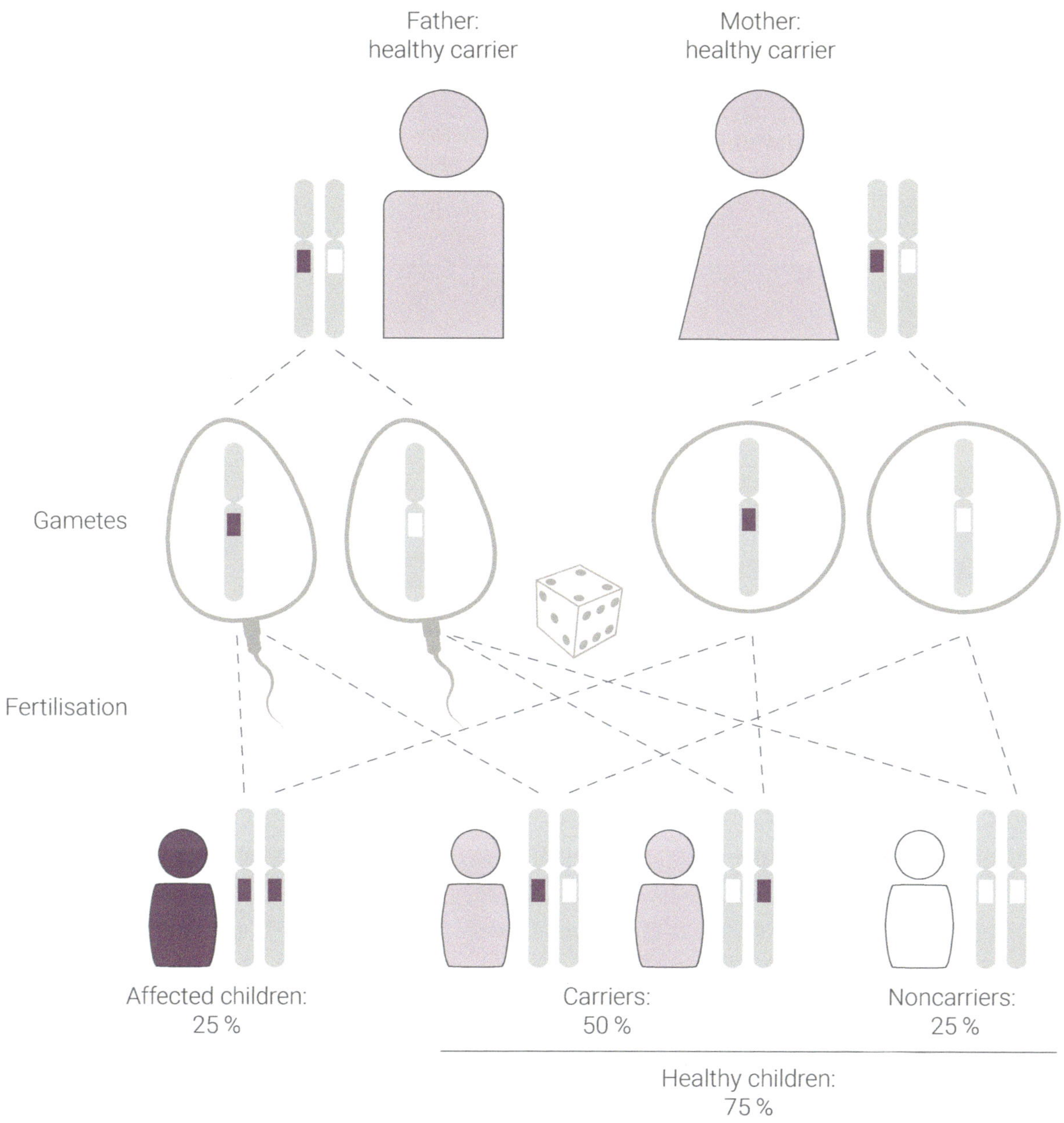

Characteristics

- Both parents are carriers:
  25 % risk of an affected child.

- Girls and boys are equally affected.

- Affected individuals commonly
  occur in one generation only.

- There is an increased risk of affected
  offspring in consanguineous marriages.

Affected children:
25 %

Carriers:
50 %

Noncarriers:
25 %

Healthy children:
75 %

Myotonic dystrophy type 1 (DM1)

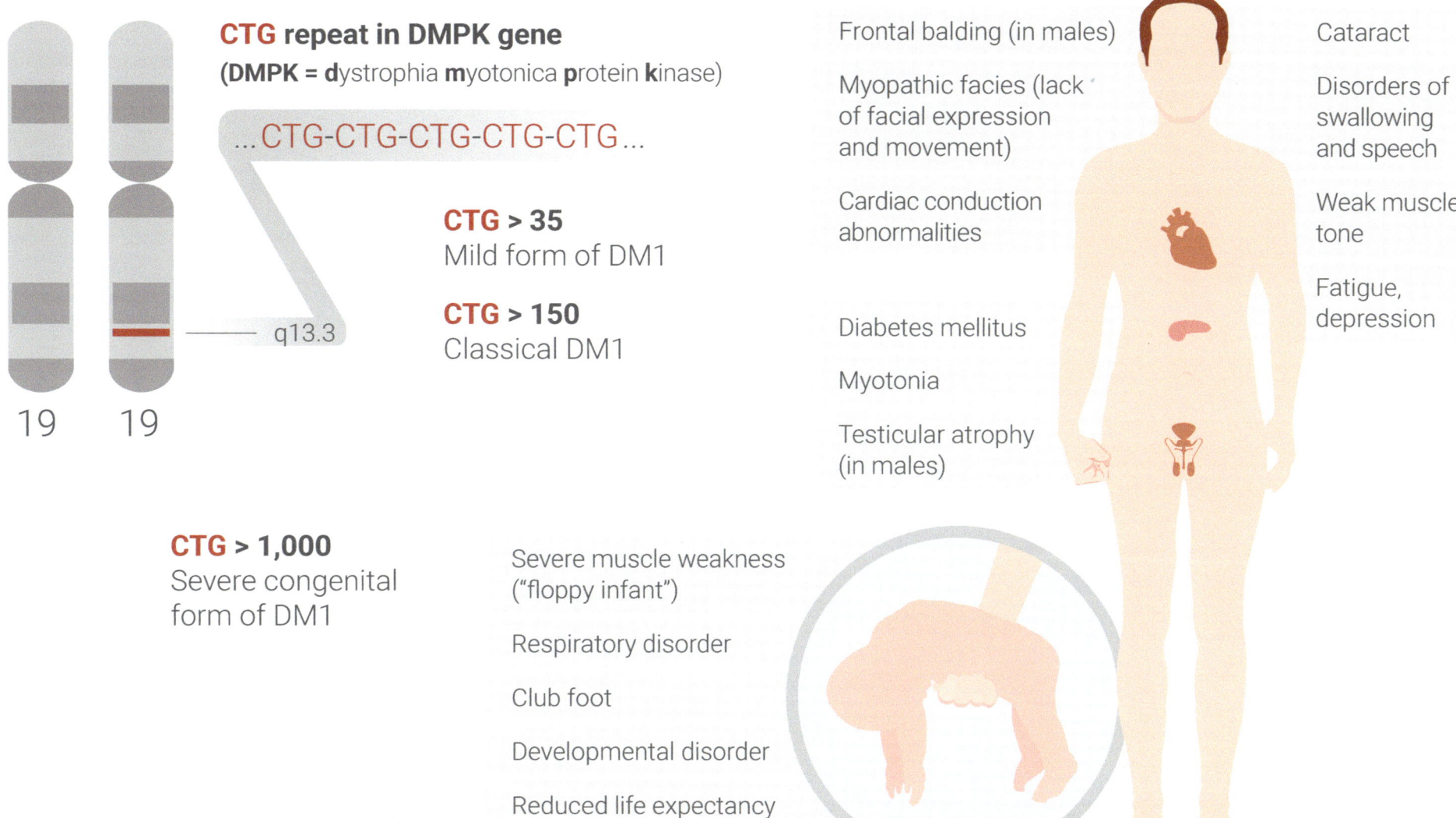

CTG repeat in DMPK gene

(**DMPK** = **d**ystrophia **m**yotonica **p**rotein **k**inase)

...CTG-CTG-CTG-CTG-CTG...

q13.3

CTG > 35
Mild form of DM1

CTG > 150
Classical DM1

19   19

CTG > 1,000
Severe congenital
form of DM1

Frontal balding (in males)

Myopathic facies (lack
of facial expression
and movement)

Cardiac conduction
abnormalities

Diabetes mellitus

Myotonia

Testicular atrophy
(in males)

Cataract

Disorders of
swallowing
and speech

Weak muscle
tone

Fatigue,
depression

Severe muscle weakness
("floppy infant")

Respiratory disorder

Club foot

Developmental disorder

Reduced life expectancy

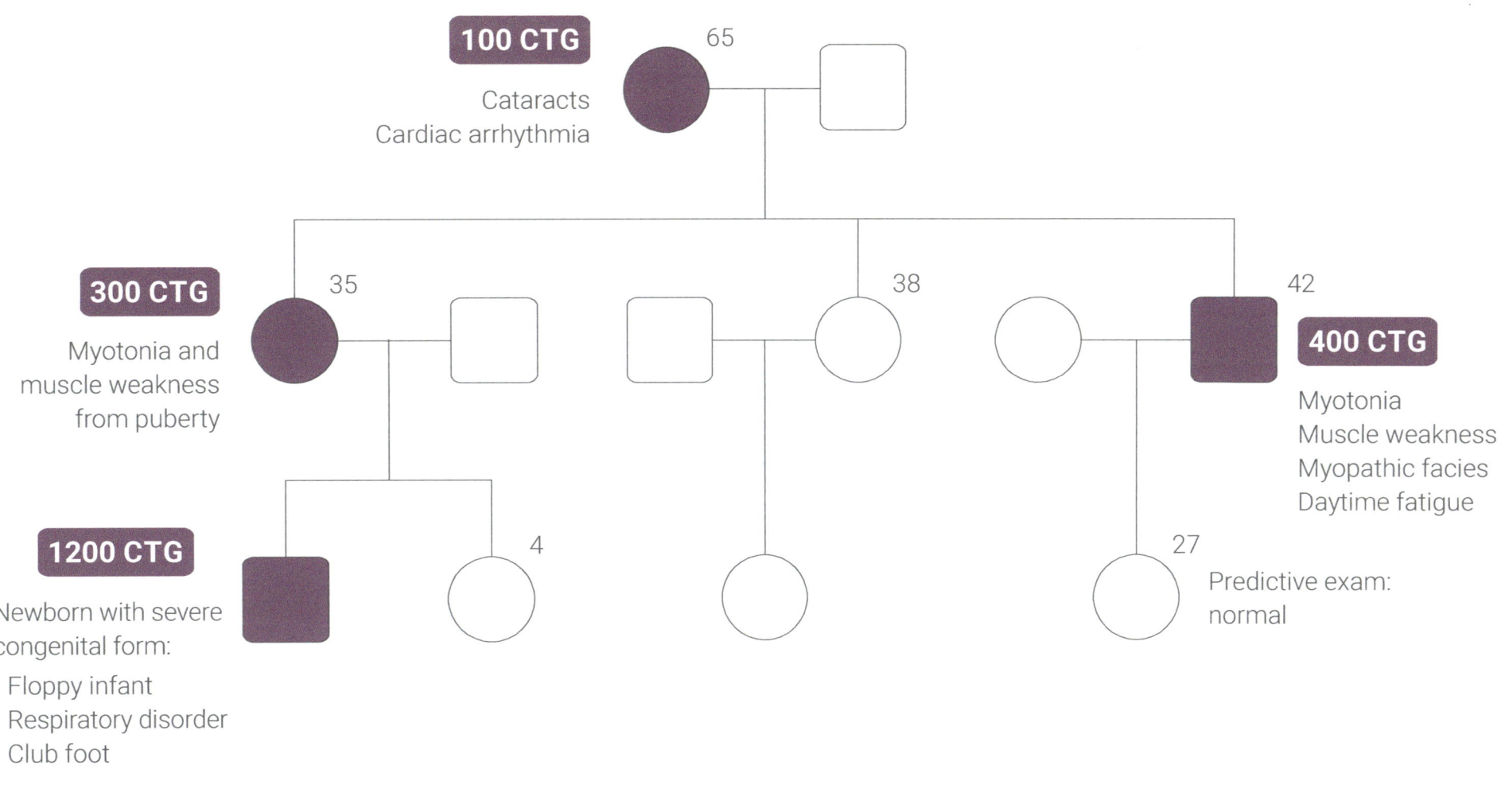

100 CTG

Cataracts
Cardiac arrhythmia

65

300 CTG

Myotonia and
muscle weakness
from puberty

35

38

42

400 CTG

Myotonia
Muscle weakness
Myopathic facies
Daytime fatigue

1200 CTG

Newborn with severe
congenital form:
• Floppy infant
• Respiratory disorder
• Club foot

4

27

Predictive exam:
normal

Healthy

Affected (DM1)

35   Age

Inheritance: autosomal dominant
Severe congenital form usually occurs only if
inherited from an affected mother (anticipation).

Huntington disease:

neurodegenerative disease
with movement disorder (chorea)
and mental symptoms,
e.g. depression and dementia

Onset: variable,
usually between age 30 and 60

Incidence:
1:10,000–20,000

Therapy: symptomatic only

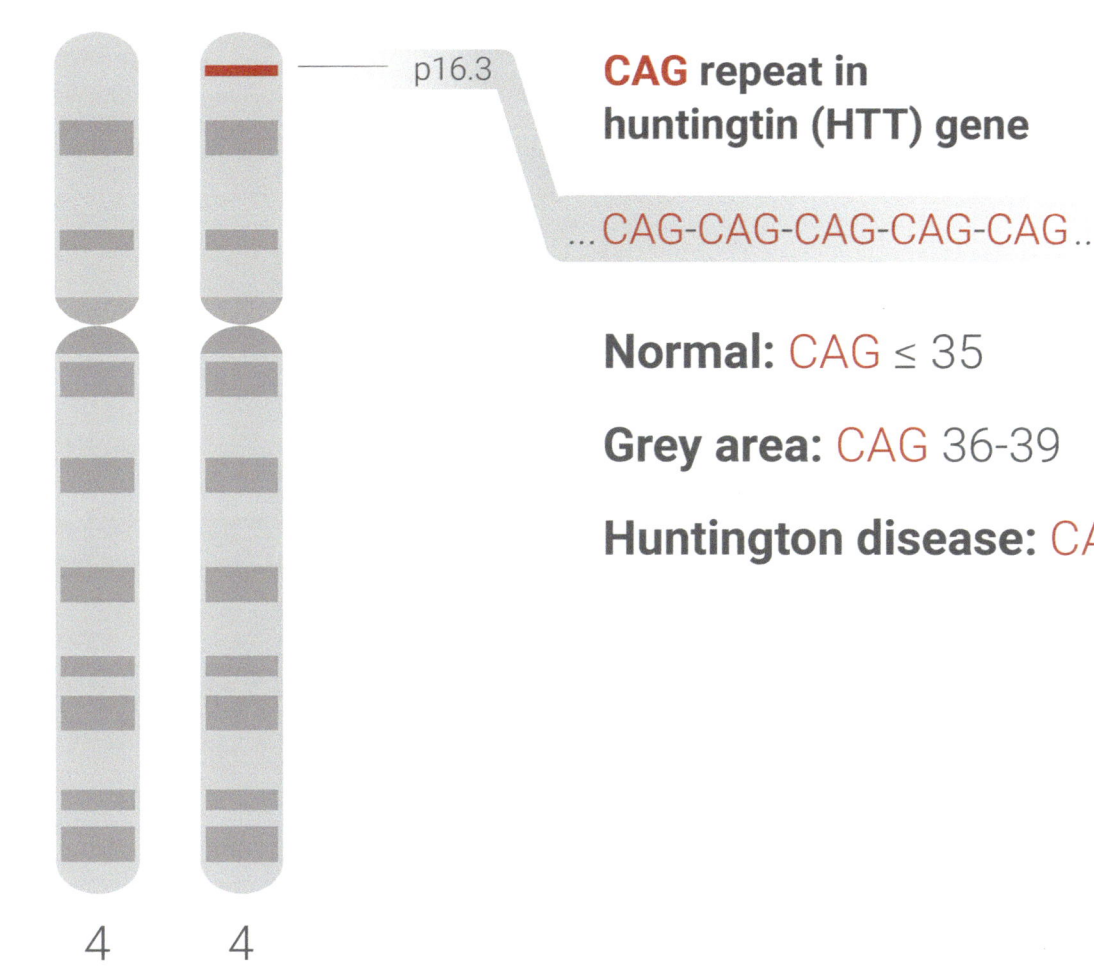

p16.3

**CAG repeat in
huntingtin (HTT) gene**

...CAG-CAG-CAG-CAG-CAG...

Normal: CAG ≤ 35

Grey area: CAG 36-39

Huntington disease: CAG ≥ 40

4   4

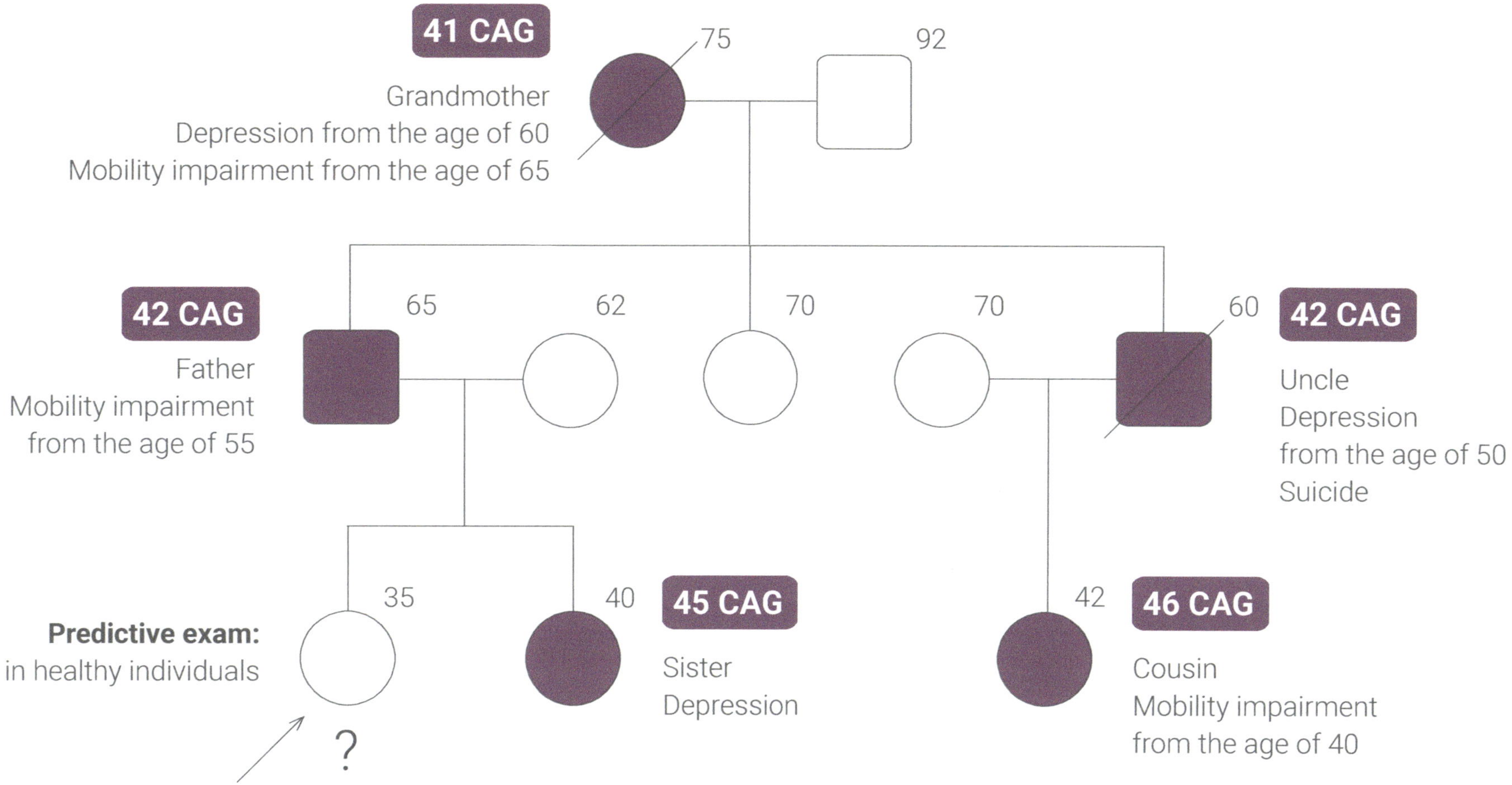

41 CAG

Grandmother
Depression from the age of 60
Mobility impairment from the age of 65

75   92

42 CAG

Father
Mobility impairment
from the age of 55

65   62   70   70   60   **42 CAG**

Uncle
Depression
from the age of 50
Suicide

Predictive exam:
in healthy individuals

35   40   **45 CAG**

Sister
Depression

?

42   **46 CAG**

Cousin
Mobility impairment
from the age of 40

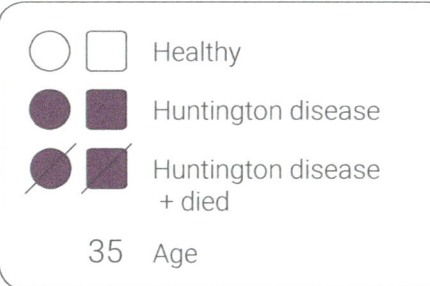

○ □ Healthy

● ■ Huntington disease

● ■ Huntington disease
   + died

35 Age

Inheritance: autosomal dominant
Anticipation: earlier symptoms in next generation
Repeat expansion: common if paternal inheritance involved

Haemophilia: two forms

	Haemophilia A	Haemophilia B
Cause	Factor VIII deficiency	Factor IX deficiency
Incidence	1:5,000 boys	1:30,000 boys

Severity grades by factor activity:

Normal:	50 – 100 %
Mild:	6 – 30 %
Moderate:	1 – 5 %
Severe:	<1 %

Therapy:

• Prophylactic administration of the missing factor
• Problem: inhibitor formation (immune response, approx. 30 %)

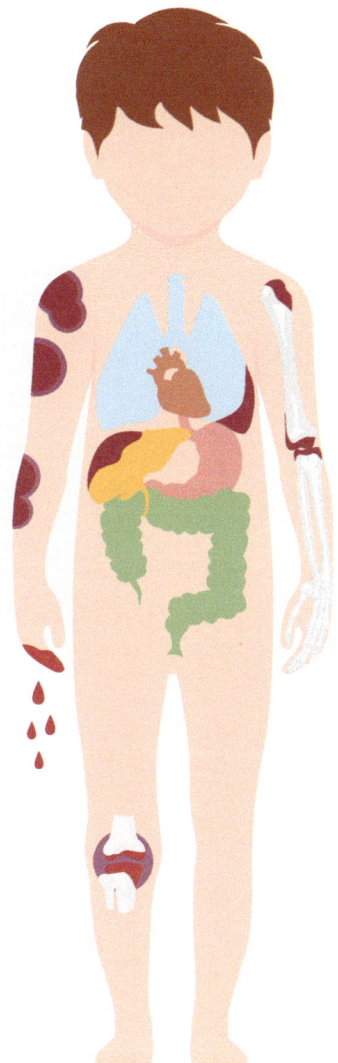

Frequent extensive bruising

Bleeding even without trauma

Bleeding into joints, muscles, internal organs and head

Long after-bleeding

Inheritance of haemophilia A and B (factor VIII/IX gene)

X-linked inheritance

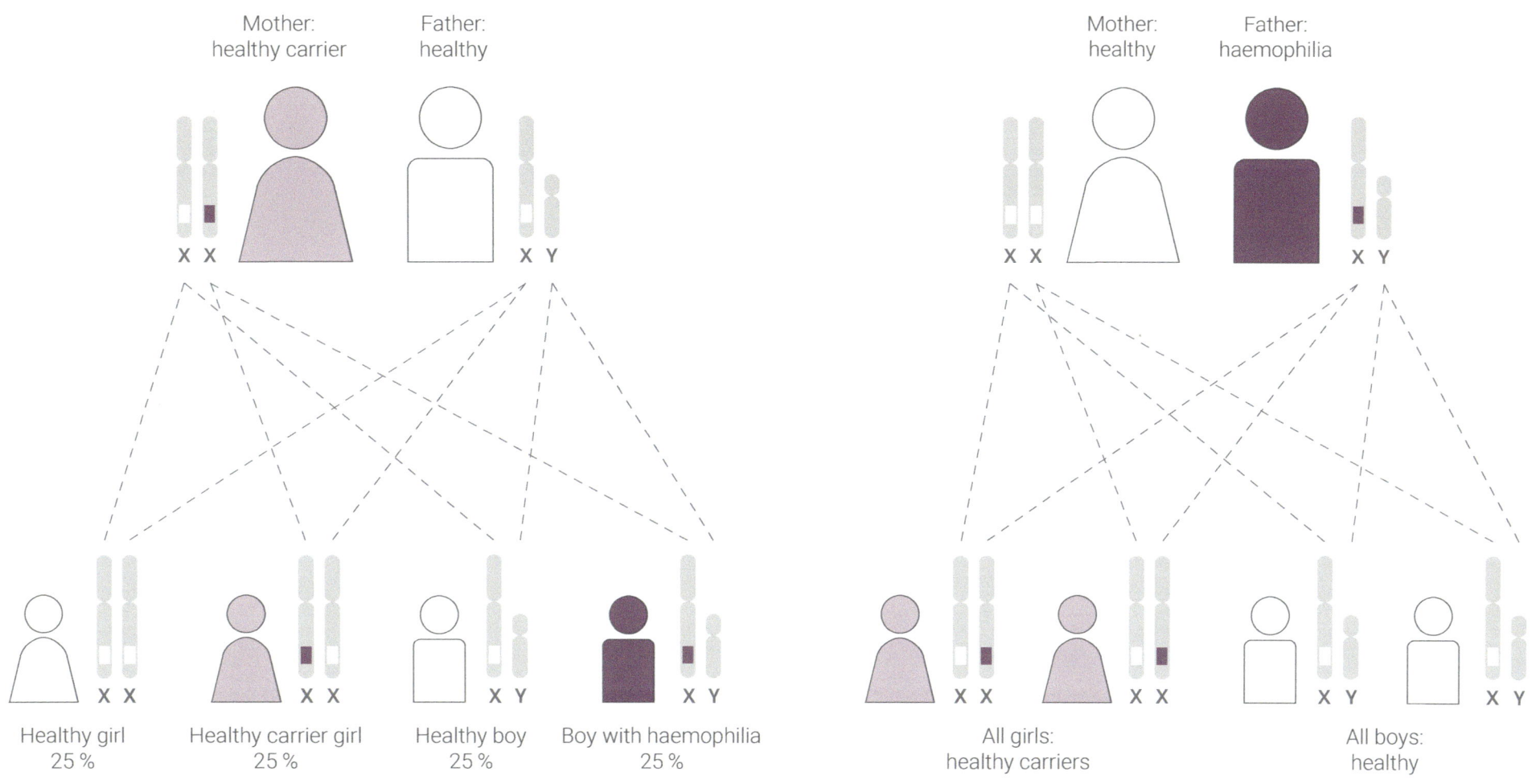

Risk factor	Prevalence in general population	Increased risk of thrombosis (relative risk)
Factor V Leiden mutation	5 % (heterozygous) 0.15 % (homozygous)	7 x (heterozygous) 26 x (homozygous)
Prothrombin mutation G20210A	3 %	3 x
Factor V Leiden and prothrombin mutation (both heterozygous)	0.14 %	36 x
Protein C deficiency	0.3 %	10–20 x
Protein S deficiency	1 %	2–20 x
Antithrombin deficiency	0.02 %	50 x
Factor VIII increased > 150 %	20 %	5 x
Anticardiolipin antibodies	11 %	3 x
Lupus anticoagulant	0.8 %	11 x

Background risk of thrombosis, age-dependent, per year:
- 20 years: 1:10,000 (0.01 %)
- 60 years: 1:1,000 (0.1 %)
- 90 years: 1:100 (1 %)

Thrombosis-promoting factors:
- Immobilisation (e.g. after surgery)
- Pregnancy
- Hormone use
- Age
- Obesity

Genetic cause: approx. 30 %

Indications for diagnostics:
- Thrombosis at a young age (< 45 years)
- Increased incidence of thrombosis in family members
- Recurrent pregnancy loss
- Before taking oral contraceptives (the pill) or hormone replacement therapy in individuals with a positive personal or family history